Medical-Surgical Nursing Test Success

Karen K. Gittings, DNP, RN, CNE, Alumnus CCRN, is an assistant professor of nursing at Francis Marion University, Florence, South Carolina. Karen received her diploma in nursing from the Washington Hospital School of Nursing and her BSN from the University of Maryland, Baltimore County campus. She received her MSN with specialization in nursing education and her DNP from Duquesne University in Pittsburgh, Pennsylvania. Karen achieved certification in online instruction in 2011. Karen has extensive experience in critical care nursing and has been a certified critical care registered nurse (CCRN) since 1991. Her areas of teaching expertise are medical-surgical nursing, critical care, and cardiac nursing. She has taught both junior- and senior-level undergraduate, baccalaureate nursing students in the classroom and clinical settings. Karen's work on the topic of nurses and body art has been published in *Nursing 2012* and *Nursing Management*. She also contributed to *Fast Facts for Developing a Nursing Academic Portfolio* (2012). Karen has also presented nationally on the topics of "Intravenous Education through Simulation" and "Developing an Effective Nurse Educator Academic Portfolio for Career Growth and Advancement." Karen is a member of Sigma Theta Tau International Honor Society of Nursing and Phi Kappa Phi. She is currently the president of the Francis Marion University Department of Nursing Honor Society and past president of the Pee Dee Area Chapter of the American Association of Critical Care Nurses. She is a recipient of multiple Outstanding Faculty Caring Teacher Awards at Francis Marion University and the South Carolina Palmetto Gold Award (2005).

Rhonda M. Brogdon, DNP, MSN, MBA, RN, is an assistant professor of nursing at Francis Marion University, Florence, South Carolina, where she is the course coordinator of nursing research in practice for prelicensure BSN students and the coordinator of the RN–BSN educational track. She has also taught health assessment for prelicensure BSN students and served as lab coordinator for the course. Previous to accepting her current teaching position, Rhonda was a part-time clinical faculty member for the Medical University of South Carolina School of Nursing/Francis Marion University Satellite Nursing Program. Dr. Brogdon earned her DNP degree from Duquesne University, Pittsburgh, Pennsylvania (2010). Dr. Brogdon's 16 years of clinical experience include renal nursing, discharge nurse–case management/counseling discharge planning, charge nurse, and medical-surgical renal staff nurse. She has contributed to *Fast Facts for Developing a Nursing Academic Portfolio* (2012), and has presented nationally on the topic. Dr. Brogdon has been the recipient of the 2007 Caring Clinical Instructor Award, Clemson Scholar of Promise (1990–1994), nominated as RN of the Year by her peers for 2 years, and was consistently evaluated as a "role model" nurse. She was awarded the African-American Faculty and Staff Coalition Diversity Award for Francis Marion University in 2013. She is currently the vice president of the Francis Marion University Nursing Honor Society.

Frances H. Cornelius, PhD, MSN, RN-BC, CNE, is associate clinical professor, chair of the MSN Advanced Practice Role Department and coordinator of informatics projects at Drexel University, College of Nursing and Health Professions. Fran has taught nursing since 1991, at several schools of nursing. She taught community health at Madonna University (Livonia, MI), Oakland (MI) University, University of Pittsburgh (PA), and Holy Family College (Philadelphia, PA). Fran taught adult health and gerontology at Widener University School of Nursing until 1997, when she began teaching at Drexel. In 2003, she was a Fellow at the Biomedical Library of Medicine. She is a certified nurse informaticist and has been the recipient of several grants. She has collaborated on the development of mobile applications as coordinator of informatics projects, including the Patient Assessment and Care Plan Development (PACPD) tool, which is a PDA tool with a Web-based companion, and Gerontology Reasoning Informatics Programs (the GRIP project). She is the coeditor (with Mary Gallagher Gordon) and chapter contributor of *PDA Connections*, an innovative textbook designed to teach health care professionals how to use mobile devices for point-of-care access of information. She is a coauthor of *Maternal-Child Nursing Test Success: An Unfolding Case Study Review* (2012); *Fundamentals of Nursing Test Success: An Unfolding Case Study Review* (2013); *Medical-Surgical Nursing Test Success: An Unfolding Case Study Review* (2013); and *Community Health Nursing Test Success: An Unfolding Case Study Review* (2013). She has written six book chapters and has published 19 journal articles on her work. She has been invited to deliver 26 presentations and has delivered more than 50 peer-reviewed presentations mostly in the United States, but also in Spain, Canada, and Korea. She is a member of the American Informatics Association, the American Nursing Informatics Association, the American Nurses Association, and the Pennsylvania State Nurses Association.

Medical-Surgical Nursing Test Success: An Unfolding Case Study Review

Karen K. Gittings, DNP, RN, CNE, Alumnus CCRN
Rhonda M. Brogdon, DNP, MSN, MBA, RN
Frances H. Cornelius, PhD, MSN, RN-BC, CNE

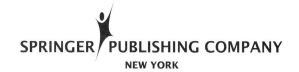

SPRINGER PUBLISHING COMPANY
NEW YORK

Springer Publishing Company, LLC
11 West 42nd Street
New York, NY 10036
www.springerpub.com

Acquisitions Editor: Margaret Zuccarini
Composition: S4Carlisle Publishing Services

ISBN: 978-0-8261-9576-0
E-book ISBN: 978-0-8261-9577-7
eResources ISBN: 978-0-8261-9425-1

A list of eResources is available from www.springerpub.com/gittings-ancillaries

13 14 15 / 5 4 3 2

The author and the publisher of this Work have made every effort to use sources believed to be reliable to provide information that is accurate and compatible with the standards generally accepted at the time of publication. Because medical science is continually advancing, our knowledge base continues to expand. Therefore, as new information becomes available, changes in procedures become necessary. We recommend that the reader always consult current research and specific institutional policies before performing any clinical procedure. The author and publisher shall not be liable for any special, consequential, or exemplary damages resulting, in whole or in part, from the readers' use of, or reliance on, the information contained in this book. The publisher has no responsibility for the persistence or accuracy of URLs for external or third-party Internet websites referred to in this publication and does not guarantee that any content on such websites is, or will remain, accurate or appropriate.

Library of Congress Cataloging-in-Publication Data

Gittings, Karen K.
  Medical-surgical nursing test success : an unfolding case study review / Karen K. Gittings, Rhonda M. Brogdon, Frances H. Cornelius.
     p. ; cm.
  Includes bibliographical references and index.
  ISBN 978-0-8261-9576-0 — ISBN 0-8261-9576-8 — ISBN 978-0-8261-9577-7 (e-book)
  I. Brogdon, Rhonda M. II. Cornelius, Frances H. III. Title.
     [DNLM: 1. Nursing Care—methods—Problems and Exercises. 2. Nursing Assessment—methods—Problems and Exercises. 3. Perioperative Nursing—methods—Problems and Exercises. WY 18.2]
  RT55
  610.73076—dc23   2013004101

Special discounts on bulk quantities of our books are available to corporations, professional associations, pharmaceutical companies, health care organizations, and other qualifying groups. If you are interested in a custom book, including chapters from more than one of our titles, we can provide that service as well.

For details, please contact:
Special Sales Department, Springer Publishing Company, LLC
11 West 42nd Street, 15th Floor, New York, NY 10036-8002
Phone: 877-687-7476 or 212-431-4370; Fax: 212-941-7842
E-mail: sales@springerpub.com

Printed in the United States of America by Bradford & Bigelow.

Dedicated to the memory of my beloved husband, Harry E. Gittings, and in honor of my parents with love, Edwin and Marilyn Learn.

Karen K. Gittings

I dedicate this book to Jordan—the sunshine in my life, my extra special blessing from God above.

Rhonda M. Brogdon

Contents

Preface

Nurses are confronted with complex patient health issues every day. As nurses, we have to be advocates for our patients and implement our critical thinking skills into action. Although health care delivery focuses on quality of patient care, recent developments on both the national and regional levels are forcing clinical quality to the forefront as a critical issue (Burke & Matthews, 2003). As nurses, we are at the forefront in detecting, correcting, and reducing adverse outcomes in patient care. With the rapid changes that are occurring in health care, the utilization of unfolding case studies will help our future nurses answer the call of providing quality care.

Unfolding case studies can be used as a guide to assess, implement, plan, educate, and evaluate the care of patients in improving the quality of patient care. The use of unfolding case studies will help student nurses "develop skills they need to analyze, organize, and prioritize in novel situations" (Batscha & Moloney, 2005, p. 387). Unfolding case studies mimic real-life situations in nursing and are situational mental models that will assist students to problem solve, actively engage, and use critical thinking techniques (Azzarello & Wood, 2006).

As a student works through the unfolding case studies, the vision of practicing as a professional nurse who is actively problem solving takes shape. The unfolding case study method assists in the development of skills that are important for NCLEX-RN® success in assessment, planning, intervention, and evaluation of patient care. The patient care content areas that are needed for NCLEX-RN success—safe and effective care, health promotion, and physiological and psychological integrity—are interwoven in an enjoyable format without the drudgery of answering multiple-choice question after question, memorizing flashcards and medical terminology definitions, or learning test-taking tricks. eResource links to additional information are positioned throughout the book. In the e-book, clicking on the link will take the student directly to that website to study additional content, which could be as interactive as watching a procedural video on YouTube. **A list of these web links and eResources is available from www.springerpub .com/gittings-ancillaries.**

The NCLEX-RN is a content-driven test and these unfolding case studies deliver medical-surgical nursing content intermingled with active learning strategies. A variety of NCLEX-style question formats are used in this book to help students assess their own learning. They include multiple-choice questions, fill-ins, hot spots, matching, true and false, prioritizing, and calculations. Questions are consistent with current NCLEX-RN testing methods.

Education is going to be the first step in adequately providing quality care that is safe and effective. Medical-surgical nursing is at the forefront of patient care as our patient population is confronted with more and more complex health decisions. The use of unfolding case studies aimed at identifying learner readiness, client needs, and client intervention will hopefully answer the call of providing quality care.

Karen K. Gittings, DNP, RN, CNE, Alumnus CCRN
Rhonda M. Brogdon, DNP, MSN, MBA, RN
Frances H. Cornelius, PhD, MSN, RN-BC, CNE

References

Azzarello, J., & Wood, D. E. (2006). Assessing dynamic mental models: Unfolding case studies. *Nurse Educator, 31*(1), 10–14.

Batscha, C., & Moloney, B. (2005). Using PowerPoint® to enhance unfolding case studies. *Journal of Nursing Education, 44*(8), 387.

Burke, F. G., & Matthews, M. (2003). *Can you corner the market on health care quality?* Retrieved from http://articles.corporate.findlaw.com/articles/file/00998

Acknowledgments

Thank you to my friend and colleague, Rhonda Brogdon; your constant friendship and encouragement made this journey possible. Thank you to my mentor and friend, Dr. Ruth Wittmann-Price, for your endless support and inspiration. Thank you to my parents and family for their unending love and belief in me. And to Harry, I know you are smiling.

—*Karen K. Gittings*

First, and foremost, I want to thank God for helping me complete this book with my colleague and friend, Karen K. Gittings. Thank you, Karen, for your support and for being my cheerleader. Second, I want to thank my parents, George and Ella Hunter, for standing beside me throughout my nursing career and while writing this book. You have been my inspiration and motivation for continuing to improve my knowledge and in moving my career forward. You have been there for me in the good and challenging times. I could not have asked for more loving parents. I love you! Next, I want to thank my husband, Edward, and my son, Jordan, for having the patience with me in taking on another endeavor, which decreased the amount of time I spent with you. In addition, I want to thank my colleagues in the Department of Nursing at Francis Marion University for your support and encouragement throughout the process of writing this book. A huge thank you to Frances Cornelius for your feedback and for being a contributing author to this book. Also, words cannot express my gratitude to my department chair and mentor, Dr. Ruth Wittmann-Price. Your knowledge throughout this process was invaluable. Your continued support and belief in me pushed me harder in wanting this book to be a success. Thank you for your long nights in reading and editing this book. You have been a role model to me since day one. Your caring and encouragement meant a lot to me. Thank you for the time you spent with Jordan so I could write. I also want to thank Springer Publishing Company for giving me this tremendous opportunity. Last, I want to thank all the patients for allowing me to be your nurse. It is truly rewarding when I know that I made a difference in your care. It is GREAT to be a NURSE!!

—*Rhonda M. Brogdon*

Nursing Test Success

With Ruth A. Wittmann-Price as Series Editor

Maternal-Child Nursing Test Success:
An Unfolding Case Study Review
Ruth A. Wittmann-Price, PhD, RN, CNS, CNE, and
Frances H. Cornelius, PhD, MSN, RN-BC, CNE

Fundamentals of Nursing Test Success:
An Unfolding Case Study Review
Ruth A. Wittmann-Price, PhD, RN, CNS, CNE, and
Frances H. Cornelius, PhD, MSN, RN-BC, CNE

Community Health Nursing Test Success:
An Unfolding Case Study Review
Frances H. Cornelius, PhD, MSN, RN-BC, CNE, and
Ruth A. Wittmann-Price, PhD, RN, CNS, CNE

Medical-Surgical Nursing Test Success:
An Unfolding Case Study Review
Karen K. Gittings, DNP, RN, CNE, Alumnus CCRN, Rhonda M. Brogdon,
DNP, MSN, MBA, RN, and Frances H. Cornelius, PhD, MSN, RN-BC, CNE

Leadership and Management in Nursing Test Success:
An Unfolding Case Study Review
Ruth A. Wittmann-Price, PhD, RN, CNS, CNE, and
Frances H. Cornelius, PhD, MSN, RN-BC, CNE

1

Nursing Care of the Patient With Cardiovascular Disease

Karen K. Gittings

Unfolding Case Study #1 ▚ Edwin

Edwin is a 56-year-old White male who was sent to his primary care provider (PCP) after his blood pressure was found to be 176/94 at a health screening at his place of employment. His blood pressure is currently 160/94. He has not previously been diagnosed with hypertension so Edwin has many questions as the nurse reviews his health history.

Exercise 1-1: *Select all that apply*
The nurse identifies the following risk factors for hypertension:

- ❏ Family history
- ❏ Age
- ❏ Dyslipidemia
- ❏ Obesity
- ❏ Smoking

The nurse completes Edwin's health history. Edwin is 5 feet 9 inches tall and 240 pounds. He has been a one pack per day (PPD) smoker for 33 years. He is employed as a supervisor at a state agency and his job is mostly sedentary. After further reviewing Edwin's health history, the nurse finds that both of Edwin's parents had hypertension and heart disease.

Exercise 1-2: *Fill-in*
Edwin has risk factors that increase his risk for future cardiac disease. Identify at least three of Edwin's risk factors. _____, _____, and _____.

eResource 1-1: Heart disease risk calculators can be utilized as an effective patient teaching tool:
- University of Maryland Heart Center: http://goo.gl/UaNIA
- MedCalc, a comprehensive library of medical calculators, available online and as "apps" for mobile devices.
  - Online: [Pathway: www.medcalc.com → select "Cardiology" → select "Heart Disease Risk" and enter patient data]
  - Mobile device: [MedCalc → select "Categories" → select "Cardiology" → select "Framingham CV Risk" and enter patient data]

Exercise 1-3: *Fill-in*

The nurse informs Edwin that in treating his hypertension, the goal is to prevent _____ and to keep his blood pressure at or lower than

_____.

 eResource 1-2: To reinforce her patient teaching, the nurse shows Edwin two brief videos:
- *Understanding High Blood Pressure—The Risks:* http://youtu.be/FrDfzlFcUT0
- *5 Major Effects of High Blood Pressure:* http://youtu.be/lCLHbwBBvFc

After Edwin is seen by the PCP, the nurse reviews the treatment regimen with Edwin, which includes: (a) weight reduction, (b) adopting the DASH diet, (c) decreasing sodium intake, (d) increasing physical activity, and (e) smoking cessation.

Exercise 1-4: *Multiple-choice question*

When educating patients about a DASH diet, the nurse includes the following information:

    A. Increase intake of fruits, vegetables, and meat products

    B. Increase intake of fruits, vegetables, and grains; lower fat intake

    C. Increase intake of low-fat dairy foods and meat products

    D. Decrease intake of fruits, vegetables, and meat products

Edwin is placed on a 2-gram sodium-restricted diet.

Exercise 1-5: *Select all that apply*

The nurse understands that the patient needs further teaching when the patient chooses the following foods when on a 2-gram sodium diet:

    ❏ Fresh fruits

    ❏ Canned vegetables

    ❏ Lunch meats

    ❏ Plain pasta

    ❏ Fast foods

Answers to this chapter begin on page 27.

eResource 1-3: To supplement dietary teaching, the nurse provides the American Heart Association's guide for Reading Food Nutrition Labels: http://goo.gl/0wY0i

In addition to lifestyle modifications, Edwin is also started on HCTZ (hydrochlorothiazide) 25 mg orally (PO) daily.

Exercise 1-6: *Fill-in*

The three electrolytes that are often lost as a result of thiazide diuretics include: _____, _____, and _____.

At Edwin's next appointment, the nurse draws a basic metabolic panel (BMP). The results are as follows:

Glucose	118 mg/dL
Sodium	139 mEq/L
Chloride	100 mEq/L
Potassium	3.2 mEq/L
Blood urea nitrogen (BUN)	12 mg/dL
Creatinine	0.9 mg/dL

Exercise 1-7: *Matching*

Match the lab test in Column A to its normal value in Column B.

Column A	Column B
A. Potassium	_____ 135–145 mEq/L
B. Chloride	_____ 3.5–5.0 mEq/L
C. Glucose	_____ 0.6–1.2 mg/dL
D. Sodium	_____ 60–110 mg/dL
E. Creatinine	_____ 7–18 mg/dL
F. BUN	_____ 97–107 mEq/L

 eResource 1-4: Web-based resources for normal blood values:
- Nursing Central: http://goo.gl/qosiq
- University of Minnesota: http://goo.gl/sTM1A

Edwin is started on potassium chloride (KCl) 20 mEq PO daily. The nurse also instructs him on foods high in potassium to include in his diet.

Exercise 1-8: *Select all that apply*

Identify which foods are rich in potassium:
- ❑ Oranges
- ❑ Strawberries
- ❑ Cheese
- ❑ Potatoes
- ❑ Chicken

Answers to this chapter begin on page 27.

Edwin is rescheduled to visit his PCP in 1 month to evaluate whether his dietary and lifestyle changes, as well as his medications, are effective for his hypertension.

Unfolding Case Study #2 ▬ Randy

Randy is a 48-year-old White male who presents to his primary care provider (PCP) with recent complaints of chest pain. The nurse further assesses Randy's complaint of chest pain to find that it is a sharp, intermittent pain occurring in the middle of his chest. The pain primarily occurs when he is exerting himself, lasts only a few minutes, and resolves after resting.

Exercise 1-9: *Fill-in*
Based on the symptoms Randy is reporting, the nurse suspects that he is experiencing

_____ .

Exercise 1-10: *Select all that apply*
Modifiable risk factors for coronary artery disease (CAD) include:

❑ Tobacco use

❑ Elevated lipid, cholesterol levels

❑ Physical inactivity

❑ Family history of CAD

❑ Diabetes

❑ Age (men older than 45 years; women older than 55 years)

❑ Obesity

The nurse completes a health history on Randy to determine if he has risk factors for coronary artery disease. In addition to his age, Randy is mildly overweight and physically inactive. There is also a significant family history of coronary artery disease.

 eResource 1-5: To supplement patient teaching regarding managing risk factors, the nurse connects Randy to the American Heart Association's Heart Risk Calculator: http://goo.gl/fHms0

After being seen by the PCP, Randy is scheduled for lab work, an electrocardiogram (ECG), and echocardiogram. He is also given a prescription for sublingual nitroglycerin (NTG) as needed (PRN).

Exercise 1-11: *Multiple-choice question*
After educating Randy on proper administration of NTG, the nurse determines that he needs further instruction when he states:

     A. "I should place the NTG tablet under my tongue and let it dissolve."

     B. "I can take one NTG tablet every 5 minutes to a maximum of three tablets."

C. "I can continue to take as many NTG tablets as needed until my chest pain is gone."

D. "I should keep my NTG tablets in their original bottle."

 eResource 1-6: To supplement your understanding of this medication, consult Medscape on your mobile device. To download the "app," go to http://goo.gl/ObHsx: [Pathway: Medscape → enter "nitroglycerin" in the search field → scroll down to select "nitroglycerin sublingual" to access content]

At his next appointment, the physician reviews Randy's lab results with him. The results are as follows:

Cholesterol 246 mg/dL

Triglycerides 154 mg/dL

LDL cholesterol 124 mg/dL

HDL cholesterol 50 mg/dL

Exercise 1-12: *Matching*
Match the lab test in Column A to its normal value in Column B.

Column A	Column B
A. Cholesterol	_____ > 60 mg/dL
B. LDL cholesterol	_____ < 150 mg/dL
C. HDL cholesterol	_____ < 200 mg/dL
D. Triglycerides	_____ < 100 mg/dL

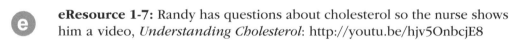 **eResource 1-7:** Randy has questions about cholesterol so the nurse shows him a video, *Understanding Cholesterol*: http://youtu.be/hjv5OnbcjE8

Randy was instructed to follow a low cholesterol diet and increase his physical activity.

eResource 1-8: To supplement patient diet teaching, the nurse shows Randy a video, *The Foods That Lower LDL*: http://youtu.be/AOcky3fUx5k

He was also given a prescription for pravastatin (Pravachol) and scheduled for a follow-up appointment in 6 months. The nurse spent time educating Randy on coronary artery disease and angina.

Exercise 1-13: *Fill-in*
Identify at least three potential adverse effects of the statin drugs:

1. _____

2. _____

3. _____

eResource 1-9: To learn more about adverse effects and precautions related to pravastatin, refer to Epocrates:
- On mobile device: [Pathway: Epocrates → select "Drugs" → enter "pravastatin" in the search field → select "pravastatin" again → view "Adverse Reactions" and "Contraindications/Cautions"]
- Online: [Pathway: https://online.epocrates.com → enter "pravastatin" in the search field → select "pravastatin" again → view "Adverse Reactions" and "Contraindications/Cautions"]

Exercise 1-14: *Fill-in*
Acute angina attacks are usually triggered by an event; common triggers include:
_____, _____,
_____, and _____.

Exercise 1-15: *Select all that apply*
Typical clinical manifestations of stable angina include:
- ❏ Pain that often occurs with exertion
- ❏ Pain that is often relieved by rest or nitrates
- ❏ Pain that occurs more often at night
- ❏ Pain that increases in severity or frequency over time
- ❏ Pain that usually lasts less than 5 minutes

Two years after his diagnosis of stable angina, Randy, who is now 50 years old, presents to the emergency department (ED) with complaints of midsternal chest pain (unrelieved by three NTG tablets), nausea, and diaphoresis. The nurse obtains vital signs and a 12-lead ECG. Analysis of the 12-lead ECG shows ST-elevation in leads II, III, and AVF. The physician diagnoses Randy with an acute inferior wall myocardial infarction (MI).

eResource 1-10: To practice interpreting ECGs:
- Visit the ECG Library: http://goo.gl/fKVd
- Play ECG Simulator: http://goo.gl/icSgp

Exercise 1-16: *Select all that apply*
Typical clinical manifestations of an acute myocardial infarction (MI) include:
- ❏ Midsternal chest pain, pressure, or tightness
- ❏ Pain that radiates to the jaw, shoulders, or arms
- ❏ Dry, warm skin with reddish color
- ❏ Anxiety or a sense of impending doom
- ❏ Nausea and vomiting

Exercise 1-17: *Fill-in*
Geriatric patients often do not exhibit typical clinical manifestations of MI, but more frequently present with the following: _____ or _____.

Answers to this chapter begin on page 27.

Exercise 1-18: *Fill-in*

In an acute MI, an area of myocardium is destroyed because of a significant imbalance between myocardial oxygen _____ and _____.

The nurse placed Randy in oxygen at 2 LPM, started two intravenous (IV) lines, and drew blood for laboratory testing. Randy is also given aspirin 325 mg PO and morphine 2 mg IV push. The nurse also starts a NTG drip at 5 mcg/min. A consult has been placed to a cardiologist for percutaneous coronary intervention (PCI).

eResource 1-11: To learn more about PCI, refer to MerckMedicus Online on your mobile device: [Pathway: www.merckmedicus.com → select "Merck Manual" → select "Merck Manual for Healthcare Professionals" → select "index" → select "P" and enter "percutaneous coronary intervention" in the search field to access and review content]

Exercise 1-19: *Multiple-choice question*

Which laboratory test is specific in diagnosing an acute MI, increases within 3 to 4 hours, and remains elevated for up to 3 weeks?

    A. White blood cells (WBCs)

    B. Troponin I

    C. Myoglobin

    D. Creatine kinase (CK)

Exercise 1-20: *Matching*

Match the drug in Column A to its indication for use in Column B.

Column A	Column B
A. Aspirin	_____ Reduces pain, anxiety, and workload of the heart
B. Morphine	_____ Dissolves thrombi in the coronary artery
C. Beta blockers	_____ Vasodilator that prevents or stops anginal attacks
D. Nitroglycerin	_____ Antiplatelet drug that suppresses platelet aggregation
E. Anticoagulants	_____ Decreases incidence of future cardiac events
F. Thrombolytics	_____ Prevents further clot formation

Exercise 1-21: *Calculation*

Order: Start NTG drip at 5 mcg/min. The NTG is mixed 50 mg in 250 mL of D5W. Calculate how fast the NTG will run in mL/hr: _____

eResource 1-12: Use MedCalc to verify your answer: [Pathway: www. medcalc.com → select "Fluids/Electrolytes" → select "IV Rate and enter information into fields]

Randy is sent to the cardiac catheterization lab where he undergoes a percutaneous transluminal coronary angioplasty (PTCA) with stent placement in the right coronary artery. He is then transferred to the coronary care unit for further care.

Exercise 1-22: *Select all that apply*

Postprocedural care following PCIs includes:

- ❑ Monitor insertion site for bleeding or hematoma
- ❑ Assess peripheral pulses every 4 hours
- ❑ Restrict fluid intake for first 8 hours
- ❑ Maintain bed rest with affected leg straight and head of bed positioned as ordered
- ❑ Encourage patient to report any chest pain

After 2 days, Randy is discharged from the hospital. The nurse provides discharge instructions related to diet, activity, medications, and follow-up care.

Exercise 1-23: *Multiple-choice question*

After educating Randy on activity recommendations for postdischarge, the nurse determines that he needs further instruction when he states:

- A. "I should gradually increase my activity duration and intensity."
- B. "I should avoid exercising in extremes of heat or cold."
- C. "If I feel fatigued, I should stop the activity and rest."
- D. "The best time for exercising is after a meal."

Unfolding Case Study #3 ▨ James

James is a 70-year-old male brought to the emergency department (ED) by ambulance with complaints of shortness of breath. Upon assessment, James has labored breathing at 36 breaths/min and tachycardia at 112 beats/min. His pulse oximetry is 90% on 40% oxygen via a face mask. Crackles are heard throughout his lungs. Jugular venous distension (JVD) is noted.

Exercise 1-24: *Fill-in*

Based on James' admission assessment, he is exhibiting clinical manifestations of

_____.

Exercise 1-25: *Select all that apply*

Potential causes of heart failure include:

- ❑ Cardiomyopathy
- ❑ Fluid overload

Answers to this chapter begin on page 27.

❏ Coronary artery disease

❏ Cardiac dysrhythmias

❏ Increased salt intake

❏ Hypertension

Exercise 1-26: *Select all that apply*

Typical signs and symptoms of heart failure include:

❏ Dyspnea on exertion

❏ Change in mental status

❏ Edema

❏ Increased urine output

❏ Weight loss

❏ Jugular venous distension

Exercise 1-27: *Multiple-choice question*

Patients in left-sided heart failure can exhibit signs of forward failure and signs of backward failure. Signs of backward failure include:

A. Dyspnea at rest, crackles, cough, and oliguria

B. Orthopnea, nocturia, confusion, and fatigue

C. Dyspnea at rest, paroxysmal nocturnal dyspnea, crackles, and cough

D. Clammy skin, fatigue, oliguria, and crackles

The physician orders a chest x-ray, ECG, arterial blood gases (ABGs), and lab work to be done. After an IV is inserted, the nurse administers furosemide (Lasix) 20 mg IV push.

e **eResource 1-13:** To learn more about furosemide, consult Skyscape's RxDrugs on your mobile device (www.skyscape.com): [Pathway: Skyscape → select "RxDrugs" → enter "lasix" into the search field → select "furosemide [IM/IV]" to review content]

The patient's medical record shows a past history of hypertension, diabetes, MI × 2, congestive heart failure (CHF), and chronic renal insufficiency.

Exercise 1-28: *Calculation*

Order: Give Lasix 20 mg IV push. Lasix is supplied 40 mg in 4 mL.

Calculate how much Lasix to administer in mL: _____

Exercise 1-29: *Fill-in*

Which lab test is a key diagnostic indicator of heart failure? _____

Exercise 1-30: *Fill-in*

Identify at least three goals for the management of patients in heart failure:

1. _____

2. _____

3. _____

James is moved to the intensive care unit (ICU). His chest x-ray shows CHF. The brain natriuretic peptide (BNP) level is 1025 pg per ml. James remains short of breath at rest. An EKG is done, which shows an ejection fraction of 40%. The physician orders James to be started on a dobutamine drip and given an additional 20 mg of IV Lasix.

> **eResource 1-14:** To learn more about dobutamine and precautions, consult Skyscape's RxDrugs on your mobile device: [Pathway: Skyscape → select "RxDrugs" → enter "dobutamine" into the search field → scroll down to view Warnings/precautions]

Exercise 1-31: *Calculation*

Order: Begin a dobutamine drip at 5 mcg/kg/min. James weighs 214 pounds. The dobutamine is supplied as 500 mg in 250 mL of D5W.

Calculate how fast to run the dobutamine in mL/hr: _____

Exercise 1-32: *Fill-in*

Arterial blood gas (ABG) results:	pH	7.47
	pO_2	82
	pCO_2	30
	HCO_3	24

Evaluate the ABG above and explain why this is occurring.

_____

_____

_____

> **eResource 1-15:** Use MedCalc's Acid–Base Online Calculator to verify your understanding: [Pathway: www.medcalc.com → select "Pulmonary" → select "ABG Calculator" and enter patient data]

James begins to diurese after the second dose of IV Lasix and his breathing begins to improve.

Exercise 1-33: *Matching*

Match the medication used to treat heart failure in Column A to its effect in Column B.

Column A	Column B
A. Benazepril	_____ Beta blocker that reduces adverse effects from constant stimulation of the sympathetic nervous system (SNS)
B. Furosemide	_____ Catecholamine that increases cardiac contractility
C. Digoxin	_____ Diuretic that removes excess extracellular fluid
D. Metoprolol	_____ Phosphodiesterase inhibitor that promotes vasodilation
E. Dobutamine	_____ Angiotensin converting enzyme (ACE) inhibitor that promotes vasodilation and diuresis
F. Milrinone	_____ Cardiac glycoside that increases the force of myocardial contraction and slows conduction through the atrioventricular (AV) node

James continues to improve and is moved to a medical floor after spending 2 days in the ICU. He is being prepared for discharge within the next 1 to 3 days.

Exercise 1-34: *Multiple-choice question*

The nurse educating James on his medications for discharge determines that he needs further instruction about his diuretic when he states:

    A. "I can hold on taking my Lasix on days that I am traveling."
    B. "I should weigh myself every day at the same time."
    C. "I should take my Lasix early in the day so I am not up all night."
    D. "I need to call the doctor if my legs start swelling more than normal."

Exercise 1-35: *Select all that apply*

Since James will be discharged on digoxin, the nurse needs to discuss which of the following signs of digoxin toxicity?

    ❑ Fatigue
    ❑ Anorexia, nausea, vomiting
    ❑ Changes in heart rate
    ❑ Changes in vision

 eResource 1-16: To learn more about digoxin and what the nurse should discuss with James, consult Skyscape's RxDrugs on your mobile device: [Pathway: Skyscape → select "RxDrugs" → enter "Digoxin" into the search field → select "Digoxin [Oral]" → scroll down to view content]

Unfolding Case Study #4 ▒ Marilyn

Marilyn is a 68-year-old female who presents to the emergency department (ED) with complaints of a fast heartbeat, chest discomfort, and shortness of breath. Initial vital signs are: heart rate 146 beats/min and irregular, respirations 26 per minute, and blood pressure 168/94.

Exercise 1-36: *Multiple-choice question*
After being connected to the heart monitor, the nurse identifies the following heart rhythm (Figure 1-1) as:

Figure 1-1: Cardiac Rhythm Strip

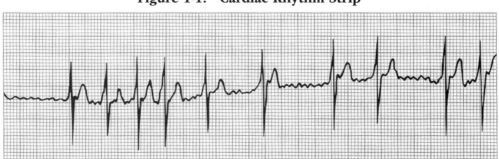

    A. Sinus tachycardia
    B. Atrial fibrillation
    C. Supraventricular tachycardia
    D. Atrial flutter

Exercise 1-37: *Matching*
Match the ECG waves, complexes, or intervals in Column A to the electrical effects in the heart in Column B.

Column A	Column B
A. T wave	_____ Early ventricular repolarization; isoelectric
B. PR interval	_____ Ventricular depolarization
C. QRS complex	_____ Atrial depolarization
D. P wave	_____ Impulse travels from sinoatrial (SA) node through atrioventricular (AV) node
E. ST segment	_____ Ventricular repolarization

 eResource 1-17: To learn more about ECG interpretation, view:
    ▪ *Intro EKG Interpretation Part 1:* http://youtu.be/ex1k_MPF-w4
    ▪ *Intro EKG Interpretation Part 2:* http://youtu.be/ecTM2O940mg

Exercise 1-38: *Fill-in*

Identify common characteristics of atrial fibrillation:

1. Ventricular rate: _____

2. Ventricular and atrial rhythm: _____

3. P waves: _____

4. Q waves: _____

5. P:QRS ratio: _____

The physician orders that the patient be given a Cardizem (diltiazem) bolus of 0.25 mg/kg and a drip started at 10 mg/hr to control the heart rate.

(e) eResource 1-18: To verify that this is a safe dose to administer, consult Epocrates on your mobile device: [Pathway: Epocrates → select "Drugs" → enter "Cardizem" into the search field → select "Adult Dosing" → scroll down to view treatment of atrial fibrillation/flutter]

Exercise 1-39: *Calculation*

Order: Give a Cardizem bolus of 0.25 mg/kg. The patient weighs 190 pounds. Begin a Cardizem drip at 10 mg/hr. The Cardizem is supplied as 125 mg in 100 mL of D5W.

Calculate the bolus to be given in mg: _____

Calculate how fast to run the Cardizem in mL/hr: _____

(e) eResource 1-19: Use MedCalc to verify your calculations:
  ▪ Online: [Pathway: www.medcalc.com → select "Fluids/Electrolytes" → select "IV Rate" and enter infusion order]
  ▪ Mobile device [MedCalc → enter "infusion" into the search field → select "Infusion Management" → enter infusion order]

After receiving the Cardizem bolus, Marilyn's heart rate begins to decrease and her chest discomfort and shortness of breath resolve. The nurse then completes a health history. Marilyn has a medical history of hypertension, coronary artery disease, hypothyroidism, and Raynaud's disease.

Exercise 1-40: *Select all that apply*

The nurse identifies that Marilyn has the following risk factors for developing atrial fibrillation:

❑ Hypertension

❑ Age

❑ Hypothyroidism

❑ Coronary artery disease

❑ Smoking

Exercise 1-41: *Select all that apply*

Patients in atrial fibrillation exhibit signs and symptoms related to a rapid heart rate and the loss of AV synchrony. Identify common signs and symptoms of atrial fibrillation.

❏ Irregular palpitations

❏ Nausea

❏ Shortness of breath

❏ Fatigue

❏ Confusion

eResource 1-20: To help Marilyn understand what atrial fibrillation is and how it is treated, the nurse shows her a video, *Atrial Fibrillation Symptoms & Treatments*: http://youtu.be/BZ1vMLPrHnk

The physician orders the following labs to be drawn: basic metabolic panel (BMP), complete blood count (CBC), magnesium, and thyroid-stimulating hormone (TSH). After being assigned an inpatient bed, Marilyn is moved to room 905 and placed on portable telemetry. All lab results are normal with the exception of the TSH level, which is below normal.

Exercise 1-42: *Fill-in*

Explain how the low TSH level may be linked to the cause of the patient's atrial fibrillation.

_____

_____

_____

_____

_____

After 24 hours, Marilyn remains in atrial fibrillation with a controlled heart rate of 84 on the Cardizem drip at 10 mg/hr. The physician orders the following new medications: Cordarone (amiodarone) 400 mg orally (PO) twice a day (BID), Coumadin (warfarin) 5 mg PO today, and restarts the Synthroid at 0.075 mg PO daily.

eResource 1-21: To verify that these drugs are safe in combination, consult Epocrates on your mobile device: [Pathway: Epocrates → select "Interaction Check" → enter all three medications and review interactions. Consider patient teaching that is warranted]

Exercise 1-43: *Fill-in*

Patients in atrial fibrillation are often started on Coumadin because of the increased risk of: _____.

Exercise 1-44: *Fill-in*

Identify the onset of action of Coumadin and the reason for this time frame.

_____

_____

_____

Exercise 1-45: *Fill-in*

In the event of overdose or excessive bleeding caused by Coumadin, the following antagonist can be given: _____.

Since Marilyn is to be discharged on Coumadin, she will require instructions on diet and monitoring of Coumadin effects/side effects.

Exercise 1-46: *Select all that apply*

Identify the vitamin K–rich foods that can antagonize the effects of Coumadin:

❑ Potatoes

❑ Broccoli

❑ Oranges

❑ Green tea

❑ Spinach

Exercise 1-47: *Multiple-choice question*

The nurse educating Marilyn on lab monitoring after discharge determines that she understands the instructions when she states:

    A. "I only need to have my labs checked every 6 months."

    B. "I have to have my partial thromboplastin time (PTT) levels checked frequently."

    C. "My international normalized ratio (INR) level should be 0.8 to 1.2 while on Coumadin."

    D. "I need to have my prothrombin time (PT) and INR levels drawn as instructed by my physician."

 eResource 1-22: To supplement the information provided to Marilyn, the nurse shows her two videos:
- ▣ *Warfarin/Coumadin Use, Part 1:* http://youtu.be/4J9luqNhEvg
- ▣ *Warfarin/Coumadin Use, Part 2:* http://youtu.be/YUVi0CXK28E

On the evening before her scheduled discharge, Marilyn is noted to have a change in her heart rhythm.

Exercise 1-48: *Multiple-choice question*

Identify the following heart rhythm (Figure 1-2):

Figure 1-2: Cardiac Rhythm Strip

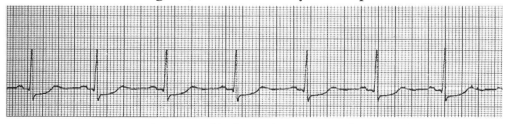

Answers to this chapter begin on page 27.

    A. Junctional rhythm

    B. Atrial flutter

    C. Sinus rhythm

    D. Sinus tachycardia

Unfolding Case Study #5 ▧ Barden

Barden is a 74-year-old male brought to the emergency department (ED) by emergency medical services personnal. He is a resident of a local nursing home. The transfer report indicates that Barden became increasingly confused over the last 2 days and is presently lethargic. His blood pressure in the nursing home was 82/46 and his heart rate was 136. On arrival to the ED, Barden's vital signs are as follows: temperature 100.2°F (oral), pulse 142, respirations 34, and blood pressure 80/50. The physician orders labs to be drawn, an IV to be started, and a Foley catheter inserted. After the Foley catheter is inserted, Barden is found to have minimal output and the urine is dark, cloudy with sediment, and foul smelling.

Exercise 1-49: *Fill-in*

Based upon the clinical manifestations that Barden is experiencing, the likely diagnosis is: _____.

Exercise 1-50: *Fill-in*

Identify three signs or symptoms that suggest this diagnosis: _____,
_____, and _____.

An hour after admission to the ED, Barden is showing no improvement. His blood pressure remains low (82/46) and his heart rate is in the 120s–130s despite IV fluids. When checking to see what laboratory tests are complete, the nurse finds that several results are coming back abnormal.

Exercise 1-51: *Fill-in*

Identify whether the following abnormal laboratory results are elevated or decreased and why they are abnormal related to Barden's case.

  1. White blood cells (WBCs) 23,000/cu mm

_____

  2. Neutrophils 80%

_____

  3. Lactic acid (venous) 22 mg/dL

_____

Answers to this chapter begin on page 27.

4. pH 7.32

_____

5. Creatinine 2.5 mg/dL

_____

(e) eResource 1-23: Web-based resources for normal blood values:
- Nursing Central: http://goo.gl/qosiq
- University of Minnesota: http://goo.gl/sTM1A

Based upon his clinical manifestations, laboratory results, and sustained hypotension, Barden is diagnosed with urosepsis and septic shock. Blood cultures $\times$ 2 are drawn and Barden is started on IV antibiotics. Orders are written for Barden to be admitted to the medical intensive care unit (MICU).

Exercise 1-52: *Fill-in*

Antibiotics orders are written with the knowledge that, traditionally, the most common causative microorganism in septic shock is: _____.

Exercise 1-53: *Matching*

Match the type of shock in Column A with its causative factors in Column B.

Column A	**Column B**
A. Hypovolemic	_____ Loss of balance between parasympathetic and sympathetic stimulation
B. Cardiogenic	_____ Widespread infection
C. Neurogenic	_____ External fluid loss or internal fluid shifts
D. Septic	_____ Severe allergic reaction
E. Anaphylactic	_____ Stress or damage to the myocardium

Exercise 1-54: *Fill-in*

Identify the three stages of shock and associated clinical findings.

Stage 1: _____

    Blood pressure: _____

    Heart rate: _____

    Respirations: _____

    Mentation:_____

    Urine output: _____

Stage 2: _____

    Blood pressure: _____

    Heart rate: _____

    Respirations: _____

    Mentation: _____

    Urine output: _____

Answers to this chapter begin on page 27.

Stage 3: _____

   Blood pressure: _____

   Heart rate: _____

   Respirations: _____

   Mentation: _____

   Urine output: _____

e   **eResource 1-24:** Consult Epocrates Online for detailed information related to evaluation and management of shock: [Pathway: https://online.epocrates.com → select "Diseases" → enter "shock" in the search field → select "septic shock" and review content]

Barden is admitted to the MICU in critical condition. His current vital signs are: temperature 100.4°F (oral), pulse 148, respirations 38, and blood pressure 78/40. Barden remains lethargic. Urine output is 10 mL/hr. An IV of 0.9% sodium chloride is infusing at 100 mL/hr and first doses of all prescribed antibiotics have been administered.

Exercise 1-55: *Fill-in*

Based on the clinical manifestations that Barden is exhibiting, he is likely in the _____ stage of shock.

Exercise 1-56: *Multiple-choice question*

When discussing urosepsis and septic shock with her orientee, the nurse identifies which common clinical manifestations?

   A. Hypotension, tachycardia, and metabolic alkalosis

   B. Cool/clammy skin, bradycardia, and metabolic acidosis

   C. Normal respirations, hypotension, and cool/clammy skin

   D. Tachycardia, decreased urine output, and metabolic acidosis

Exercise 1-57: *Select all that apply*

Identify therapies used in the treatment of septic shock:

   ❑ Fluid replacement

   ❑ Progressive activity

   ❑ Vasoactive drugs

   ❑ Nutritional support

   ❑ Early antibiotics

   ❑ Aggressive hypothermia

Barden remains hypotensive and tachycardic. The physician orders norepinephrine (Levophed) to be started to support and improve Barden's blood pressure.

e   **eResource 1-25:** To learn more about norepinephrine, consult Skyscape's RxDrugs on your mobile device: [Pathway: Skyscape → select "RxDrugs" → enter "norepinephrine" into the search field → review content]

Answers to this chapter begin on page 27.

Exercise 1-58: *Calculation*

Order: Begin a Levophed drip at 2 mcg/min. The Levophed is supplied as 4 mg in 500 mL of D5W.

Calculate how fast to run the Levophed in mL/hr: _____

> **e** **eResource 1-26:** Use MedCalc to verify your answer: [Pathway: www .medcalc.com → select "Fluids/Electrolytes" → select "IV Rate" and enter information into fields]

Barden's two daughters arrive at the hospital; they are clearly anxious and apprehensive about their father's condition. Since they have many questions, the physician has been called to update them on their father's medical status.

Exercise 1-59: *Multiple-choice question*

In dealing with patients and families who are facing critical illness and potential death, it is important for the nurse to:

    A. Reassure the patient and family that everything will be okay

    B. Maintain a strict visitation schedule

    C. Speak in a calm, reassuring voice using touch as appropriate

    D. Provide long, detailed explanations

Unfolding Case Study #6 ▧ Marcey

Marcey is a 58-year-old female who presents to her primary care provider (PCP) with complaints of pain when walking. Marcey states that she develops a cramp-like pain in her legs when walking a distance or with sustained activity that involves walking. Her past medical history includes one pack per day (PPD) smoking of cigarettes for 40 years, hypertension, and dyslipidemia. She is overweight at 5 feet 4 inches and 190 pounds.

Exercise 1-60: *Fill-in*

Taking into account Marcey's current complaint and her past medical history, the nurse determines that Marcey is likely experiencing _____ related to _____.

Exercise 1-61: *Select all that apply*

Identify physical assessment changes that can be seen as a result of inadequate arterial blood flow to the extremities:

    ❑ Loss of hair

    ❑ Decreased or absent pulses

    ❑ Severe edema

    ❑ Cool, pale skin

    ❑ Ulcers near the medial malleolus

    ❑ Rubor when extremities are dependent

Answers to this chapter begin on page 27.

The physician orders an ankle-brachial index (ABI) to be done in the office. The results are as follows:

Right brachial 140 mm Hg	Left brachial 135 mm Hg
Right dorsalis pedis 90 mm Hg	Left dorsalis pedis 80 mm Hg
Right posterior tibial 80 mm Hg	Left posterior tibial 70 mm Hg

Exercise 1-62: *Calculation*
Calculate the ABI for each foot by dividing the highest ankle systolic pressure by the higher of the two brachial systolic pressures.

Right ABI = _____

Left ABI = _____

e **eResource 1-27:** To check your calculations, use Skyscape's Archimedes on your mobile device: [Pathway: Archimedes → enter "ABI" into search field and enter patient data]

e **eResource 1-28:** To learn more about Ankle-Brachial Index Measurement, go to Medscape: [Pathway: www.medscape.org → Under the tab "Reference," select "References & Tools" → enter "ABI" into the search field → select "overview," "periprocedural care," and view the multimedia presentation of the procedure]

Marcey is diagnosed with peripheral arterial insufficiency. The nurse educates Marcey on her disease process and together they identify her risk factors. Marcey receives further instruction on how her risk can be modified.

e **eResource 1-29:** Consult Epocrates Online for detailed information related to Marcey's presentation:
- Diagnostic Tests: [Pathway: https://online.epocrates.com → select "Diseases" → enter "peripheral vascular disease" in the search field → under "Diagnosis" select "Tests" and review content]
- Treatment and prevention for Marcey: [Pathway: https://online .epocrates.com → select "Diseases" → enter "peripheral vascular disease" in the search field → under "Treatment" select and review "Tx Details," "Emerging Tx and "Prevention," and review content]

Exercise 1-63: *Select all that apply*
Identify the modifiable risk factors associated with peripheral arterial disease:
- ❑ Age
- ❑ Nicotine use
- ❑ Familial predisposition
- ❑ Sedentary lifestyle
- ❑ Hypertension
- ❑ Stress

Answers to this chapter begin on page 27.

Exercise 1-64: *Fill-in*
Marcey has several risk factors for peripheral arterial disease that further increase her risk of future heart disease. Identify those risk factors that are modifiable. _____, _____, _____, and _____.

Exercise 1-65: *Multiple-choice question*
The nurse educating Marcey on risk factor modification determines that she understands the instructions when she states:
    A. "I have been smoking a long time, but I will try to cut back some."
    B. "I need to alter my diet to reduce my calories, fat, and cholesterol intake."
    C. "If I change my diet, I can stop taking my cholesterol medication."
    D. "I need to cut back on my activity and avoid all exercise."

eResource 1-30: To help Marcey, the nurse provides additional resources for risk reduction:
■ Smokefree.gov mobile smoking cessation apps: http://smokefree.gov/apps
■ CDC's Podcast, *Smoking and Older Adults*: http://goo.gl/EjKu5

Four weeks later, Marcey is back at her PCP for follow-up and further education. She has enrolled in a smoking cessation program, and is compliant with her medication regime, but she continues to experience pain with prolonged activity associated with walking. Marcey expresses interest in learning more about diet and weight loss and strategies to better manage her disease process.

Exercise 1-66: *True or false*
Identify whether the following statements are true or false:
_____ 1. People with peripheral arterial insufficiency should position the affected extremity below the level of the heart to improve circulation.
_____ 2. Elevating the head of the bed on 6-inch blocks will improve arterial circulation.
_____ 3. People with peripheral arterial insufficiency should continue exercising even with pain in the affected extremity.

Exercise 1-67: *Select all that apply*
Identify interventions effective in promoting vasodilation and/or preventing compression:
❑ Avoid cold temperatures
❑ Use heating pads or hot water bottles on affected extremities
❑ Avoid crossing legs
❑ Avoid tight clothing
❑ Encourage stress management

Exercise 1-68: *Fill-in*
Briefly explain how nicotine negatively affects people with peripheral arterial disease.

_____

_____

e **eResource 1-31:** To further explain the effects of nicotine on the body, the nurse shows Marcey a video, *Nicotine & Smoking Facts: How Do Cigarettes Affect the Body?* http://youtu.be/YtodWKFfYjw

Exercise 1-69: *Multiple-choice question*
The nurse educating Marcey on methods for protecting her extremities determines that she needs further instruction when she states:
   A. "I should check my feet every day and notify my physician of any problems."
   B. "When my feet get dry and scaly, I rub them with a hard-bristled brush."
   C. "I should wear well-fitting shoes or slippers at all times."
   D. "I should avoid using lotion between my toes."

Marcey is able to successfully manage her disease for 4 years before the symptoms worsen. She now reports a persistent pain in her forefoot that is worse at night. Her dorsalis pedis pulses are only found with a Doppler. She is scheduled for an arteriogram of the lower extremities.

Exercise 1-70: *Fill-in*
Identify at least four complications that can occur with an arteriogram:
_____, _____,
_____, and _____.

Exercise 1-71: *Select all that apply*
Identify the nursing interventions appropriate for the care of a patient post arteriogram:
   ❑ Assess peripheral pulses in the affected extremity beginning at every 15 minutes
   ❑ Monitor insertion site for bleeding or hematoma
   ❑ Keep head of bed higher than 30 degrees
   ❑ Limit oral fluid intake
   ❑ Assess temperature and color of affected extremity

Unfolding Case Study #7 ▬ Margaret

Margaret is a 67-year-old female who presents to the emergency department (ED) with complaints of pain and swelling in her right calf. The triage nurse assesses Margaret and finds that her right lower leg is edematous, reddened, and warm to the touch. Margaret has a past medical history of hypertension, diabetes, and

Answers to this chapter begin on page 27.

osteoarthritis. She is 1 month post right knee replacement, and she reports that she is having difficulty regaining her presurgical activity level. Margaret is 5'4" and 197 pounds.

Exercise 1-72: *Fill-in*

After completing her assessment and reviewing Margaret's chief complaint and past medical/surgical history, the nurse suspects that she has:

_____

Exercise 1-73: *Fill-in*

Virchow's triad is believed to play a significant role in the development of venous thromboembolism (VTE). List the three factors that comprise Virchow's triad:

1. _____
2. _____
3. _____

 eResource 1-32: To learn more about VTE and its treatment, visit Medscape:
- Online: [Pathway: www.medscape.org → Under the tab "Reference," select "References & Tools" → enter "Deep Venous Thrombosis" into the search field → review content]
- On your mobile device: [Pathway: Medscape → enter "Deep Venous Thrombosis" into the search field → review content]

Exercise 1-74: *Fill-in*

Briefly identify Margaret's risk factors for developing deep vein thrombosis and then connect them with the factors of Virchow's triad.

1. _____
2. _____
3. _____
4. _____

Margaret is sent for a Doppler ultrasound of both legs, which confirms the diagnosis of a right leg deep vein thrombosis. The physician writes orders to admit Margaret to a medical unit and to begin enoxaparin (Lovenox) 1 mg/kg subcutaneously every 12 hours. Prior to beginning the Lovenox, the nurse draws blood per the anticoagulant protocol.

Exercise 1-75: *Select all that apply*

Identify which laboratory tests must be checked prior to beginning Lovenox and then monitored during the course of therapy:

❏ Platelets
❏ Potassium
❏ D-dimer
❏ Hemoglobin/hematocrit
❏ Activated partial thromboplastin time (aPTT)

Answers to this chapter begin on page 27.

eResource 1-33: Consult Epocrates on your mobile device to review safety and monitoring guidelines: [Pathway: Epocrates → enter "Lovenox" into search field → select "Safety/Monitoring." Also review Contraindications/ Cautions as well as Adverse Reactions]

Margaret is admitted to a medical unit. She begins asking questions about her disease process and how it could have been prevented. As the nurse works to admit Margaret, she also answers questions and begins to educate Margaret on her diagnosis.

 eResource 1-34: Consult EpocratesOnline to review content related to prevention: [Pathway: https://online.epocrates.com → select the "Diseases" tab and enter "Deep Vein Thrombosis" into the search field → Under "Treatment" select "Prevention." Also review Patient Teaching which is located under "Follow-Up"]

Exercise 1-76: *Select all that apply*
Identify clinical manifestations associated with deep vein thrombosis:

❏ Warmth in the calf area

❏ Edema

❏ Functional impairment

❏ Absence of dorsalis pedis pulse

❏ Differences in leg circumference bilaterally

Exercise 1-77: *Fill-in*
Briefly explain how Homans' sign is performed and how it is used to assess for deep vein thrombosis:

_____

_____

_____

Exercise 1-78: *True or false*
Identify whether the following statements about prevention of deep vein thrombosis are true or false:

_____ 1. Antiembolism stockings are ineffective in preventing deep vein thrombosis.

_____ 2. Early mobilization after surgery is an effective prevention therapy.

_____ 3. Low-molecular-weight heparin is an effective prophylaxis used after certain surgeries.

Answers to this chapter begin on page 27.

The nurse prepares to administer Margaret's first dose of Lovenox. It is important that Margaret receives first-dose teaching about the Lovenox as well as information that she will need in the event she goes home on this drug. It is anticipated that Margaret will also be started on warfarin (Coumadin) and discharged home in 1 to 3 days.

Exercise 1-79: *Calculation*
Order: Give enoxaparin (Lovenox) 1 mg/kg subcutaneously every 12 hours. The patient's weight is 197 pounds.
Calculate the dose of Lovenox to be given in mg: _____

Exercise 1-80: *Multiple-choice question*
The nurse educating Margaret on the action of Lovenox determines that she understands the information when she states that Lovenox will:
  A. "Dissolve the clot in my leg and prevent new ones from forming."
  B. "Prevent the clot in my leg from getting bigger and prevent new ones from forming."
  C. "Prevent the clot in my leg from getting bigger and eventually dissolve it."
  D. "Cause the clot in my leg to move and break apart."

Exercise 1-81: *Hot spot*
Mark the areas (Figure 1-3) where you would administer the Lovenox:

Figure 1-3: Abdomen

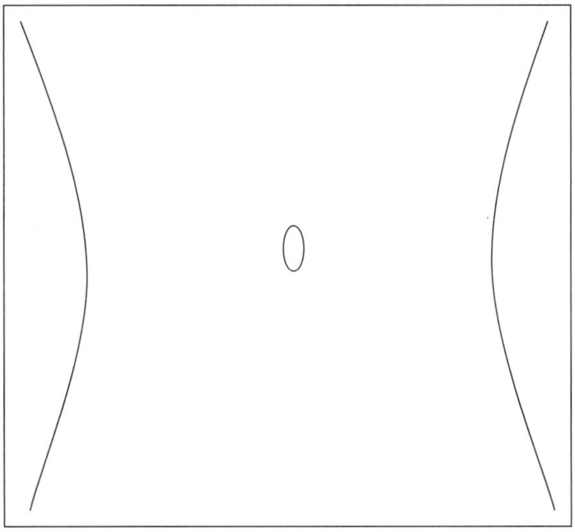

Margaret is started on warfarin (Coumadin) therapy on her second inpatient day. Three days later, her PT and INR levels are not yet therapeutic, but the physician has decided to discharge her home on Lovenox and Coumadin. Plans are for her Coumadin dose to be regulated as an outpatient, and Margaret will remain on the Lovenox until her PT and INR levels are therapeutic. Margaret receives further discharge instructions on her medications, activity level, and follow-up care.

Answers to this chapter begin on page 27.

Exercise 1-82: *Multiple-choice question*
The nurse educating Margaret on her medications for discharge determines that she needs further instruction about Lovenox when she states:
  A. "I should notify the physician if I see any blood in my urine."
  B. "I should avoid giving my Lovenox in the same location every day."
  C. "I am at increased risk for bleeding while on Lovenox and Coumadin."
  D. "I have to have my aPTT monitored every day while on Lovenox."

Exercise 1-83: *Select all that apply*
Since Margaret has been on anticoagulants for 3 days, what activities would you recommend that she continue at home?
  ❑ Elevate her right leg when recumbent
  ❑ Begin walking on a treadmill as soon as possible
  ❑ Progressively increase her ambulation
  ❑ Repetitively dorsiflex both feet when recumbent
  ❑ Keep her knees bent when sitting in the recliner

Exercise 1-84: *Matching*
Match the arterial or venous insufficiency in Column A with its typical characteristics in Column B. Answers in Column A can be used more than once.

Column A	Column B
A. Arterial insufficiency	_____ Aching, cramping type pain
B. Venous insufficiency	_____ Skin thickened, tough, and pigmented
	_____ Pulses diminished or absent
	_____ Edema moderate to severe
	_____ Ulcers usually on tips of toes or heels
	_____ Often very painful

Answers to this chapter begin on page 27.

Answers

Exercise 1-1: *Select all that apply*

The nurse identifies the following risk factors for hypertension:

☒ **Family history—YES, there is a genetic factor to hypertension.**

☒ **Age—YES, incidence of hypertension increases with age.**

☐ Dyslipidemia—NO

☒ **Obesity—YES, there is more hypertension in obese patients.**

☐ Smoking—NO

Exercise 1-2: *Fill-in*

Edwin has risk factors that increase his risk for future cardiac disease. Identify at least three of Edwin's risk factors.

Age, **smoking**, **obesity**, **physical inactivity**, and/or **family history.**

Exercise 1-3: *Fill-in*

The nurse informs Edwin that in treating his hypertension, the goal is to prevent **complications and death** and to keep his blood pressure at or lower than **140/90 mm Hg.**

Exercise 1-4: *Multiple-choice question*

When educating patients about a DASH diet, the nurse includes the following information:

A. Increase intake of fruits, vegetables, and meat products—NO, meats contain fats in large amounts.

B. **Increase intake of fruits, vegetables, and grains—YES, this is a lower fat intake.**

C. Increase intake of low-fat dairy foods and meat products—NO

D. Decrease intake of fruits, vegetables, and meat products—NO, patients should increase fruits and vegetables.

Exercise 1-5: *Select all that apply*

The nurse understands that the patient needs further teaching when the patient chooses the following foods when on a 2-gram sodium diet:

☐ Fresh fruits—NO

☒ **Canned vegetables—YES, canned vegetables use sodium to keep them fresh; choose fresh vegetables when possible.**

☒ **Lunch meats—YES, lunch meat has lots of sodium.**

❑ Plain pasta—NO

☒ **Fast foods—YES, fast food is made with sodium.**

Exercise 1-6: *Fill-in*

The three electrolytes that are often lost as a result of thiazide diuretics include: **sodium**, **potassium**, and **magnesium.**

Exercise 1-7: *Matching*

Match the lab test in Column A to its normal value in Column B.

Column A	Column B	
A. Potassium	**D**	35–145 mEq/L
B. Chloride	**A**	3.5–5.0 mEq/L
C. Glucose	**E**	0.6–1.2 mg/dL
D. Sodium	**C**	60–110 mg/dL
E. Creatinine	**F**	7–18 mg/dL
F. BUN	**B**	97–107 mEq/L

Exercise 1-8: *Select all that apply*

Identify which foods are rich in potassium:

☒ **Oranges—YES**

☒ **Strawberries—YES**

❑ Cheese—NO

☒ **Potatoes—YES**

❑ Chicken—NO

Exercise 1-9: *Fill-in*

Based on the symptoms Randy is reporting, the nurse suspects that he is experiencing **stable angina.**

Exercise 1-10: *Select all that apply*

Modifiable risk factors for coronary artery disease (CAD) include:

☒ **Tobacco use—YES**

☒ **Elevated lipid, cholesterol levels—YES**

☒ **Physical inactivity—YES**

❑ Family history of CAD—NO

☒ **Diabetes—YES**

❑ Age (men older than 45 years; women older than 55 years)—NO

☒ **Obesity—YES**

Exercise 1-11: *Multiple-choice question*

After educating Randy on proper administration of NTG, the nurse determines that he needs further instruction when he states:

A. "I should place the NTG tablet under my tongue and let it dissolve."—NO, do not swallow or chew NTG.

B. "I can take one NTG tablet every 5 minutes to a maximum of three tablets."—NO

C. "I can continue to take as many NTG tablets as needed until my chest pain is gone."—YES, only three NTG tablets should be taken for a single episode of chest pain.

D. "I should keep my NTG tablets in their original bottle."—NO

Exercise 1-12: *Matching*

Match the lab test in Column A to its normal value in Column B.

Column A	Column B	
A. Cholesterol	__C__	> 60 mg/dL
B. LDL cholesterol	__D__	< 150 mg/dL
C. HDL cholesterol	__A__	< 200 mg/dL
D. Triglycerides	__B__	< 100 mg/dL

Exercise 1-13: *Fill-in*

Identify at least three potential adverse effects of the statin drugs:

1. **Gastrointestinal problems**
2. **Myopathy**
3. **Hepatotoxicity**
4. **Peripheral neuropathy**
5. **Headache**
6. **Rash**

Exercise 1-14: *Fill-in*

Acute angina attacks are usually triggered by an event; common triggers include: **Physical exertion, cold exposure, eating a heavy meal,** and **stress or strong emotional situations.**

Exercise 1-15: *Select all that apply*

Typical clinical manifestations of stable angina include:

☒ **Pain that often occurs with exertion—YES, pain is more predictable.**

☒ **Pain that is often relieved by rest or nitrates—YES**

❑ Pain that occurs more often at night—NO, usually occurs with exertion.

❑ Pain that increases in severity or frequency over time—NO, this is a warning!

☒ **Pain that usually lasts less than 5 minutes—YES**

Exercise 1-16: *Select all that apply*

Typical clinical manifestations of an acute myocardial infarction (MI) include:

☒ **Midsternal chest pain, pressure, or tightness—YES**

☒ **Pain that radiates to the jaw, shoulders, or arms—YES, usually the left arm.**

❑ Dry, warm skin with reddish color—NO, diaphoresis and pallor common.

☒ **Anxiety—YES, patients may have a sense of impending doom.**

☒ **Nausea and vomiting—YES**

Exercise 1-17: *Fill-in*

Geriatric patients often do not exhibit typical clinical manifestations, but more frequently present with the following: **dyspnea** or **fatigue.**

Exercise 1-18: *Fill-in*

In an acute MI, an area of myocardium is destroyed because of a significant imbalance between myocardial oxygen **supply** and **demand.**

Exercise 1-19: *Multiple-choice question*

Which laboratory test is specific in diagnosing an acute MI, increases within 3 to 4 hours, and remains elevated for up to 3 weeks:

A. White blood cells (WBCs)—NO, not specific to cardiac muscle.

B. Troponin I—YES, specific for cardiac muscle.

C. Myoglobin—NO, found in cardiac and skeletal muscle.

D. Creatine kinase (CK)—NO, found in cardiac and skeletal muscle and brain tissue.

Exercise 1-20: *Matching*

Match the drug in Column A to its indication for use in Column B.

Column A		Column B
A. Aspirin	**B**	Reduces pain, anxiety, and workload of the heart
B. Morphine	**F**	Dissolves thrombi in the coronary artery
C. Beta blockers	**D**	Vasodilator that prevents or stops anginal attacks
D. Nitroglycerin	**A**	Antiplatelet drug that suppresses platelet aggregation
E. Anticoagulants	**C**	Decreases incidence of future cardiac events
F. Thrombolytics	**E**	Prevents further clot formation

Exercise 1-21: *Calculation*

Order: Start NTG drip at 5 mcg/min. The NTG is mixed 50 mg in 250 mL of D5W. Calculate how fast the NTG will run in mL/hour: **3.3 mL/hr**

Exercise 1-22: *Select all that apply*

Postprocedural care following percutaneous coronary interventions includes:

☒ **Monitor insertion site for bleeding or hematoma—YES, initially every 15 minutes.**

❑ Assess peripheral pulses every 4 hours—NO, pulses are initially checked every 15 minutes.

❑ Restrict fluid intake for first 8 hours—NO, encourage fluid intake to flush the dye out.

☒ **Maintain bed rest with affected leg straight and head of bed positioned as ordered—YES, restrictions are specified by the cardiologist.**

☒ **Encourage patient to report any chest pain—YES**

Exercise 1-23: *Multiple-choice question*

After educating Randy on activity recommendations for postdischarge, the nurse determines that he needs further instruction when he states:

A. "I should gradually increase my activity duration and intensity."—NO

B. "I should avoid exercising in extremes of heat or cold."—NO

C. "If I feel fatigued, I should stop the activity and rest."—NO

D. **"The best time for exercising is after a meal."—YES, avoid physical exercise immediately after a meal.**

Exercise 1-24: *Fill-in*

Based on James' admission assessment, he is exhibiting clinical manifestations of: **heart failure.**

Exercise 1-25: *Select all that apply*

Potential causes of heart failure include:

☒ **Cardiomyopathy—YES**

❑ Fluid overload—NO

☒ **Coronary artery disease—YES**

☒ **Cardiac dysrhythmias—YES**

❑ Increased salt intake—NO

☒ **Hypertension—YES**

Exercise 1-26: *Select all that apply*

Typical signs and symptoms of heart failure include:

☒ **Dyspnea on exertion—YES**

☒ **Change in mental status—YES**

☒ **Edema—YES**

☐ Increased urine output—NO, urine output will decrease.

☐ Weight loss—NO, weight gain occurs with fluid retention.

☒ **Jugular venous distension—YES**

Exercise 1-27: *Multiple-choice question*

Patients in left-sided heart failure can exhibit signs of forward failure and signs of backward failure. Signs of backward failure include:

A. Dyspnea at rest, crackles, cough, and oliguria—NO, oliguria is forward.

B. Orthopnea, nocturia, confusion, and fatigue—NO, nocturia, confusion, and fatigue are forward.

C. **Dyspnea at rest, paroxysmal nocturnal dyspnea, crackles, and cough—YES**

D. Clammy skin, fatigue, oliguria, and crackles—NO, clammy skin, fatigue, and oliguria are forward.

Exercise 1-28: *Calculation*

Order: Give Lasix 20 mg IV push. Lasix is supplied 40 mg in 4 mL.

Calculate how much Lasix to administer in mL: **2 mL**

Exercise 1-29: *Fill-in*

Which lab test is a key diagnostic indicator of heart failure? **BNP**

Exercise 1-30: *Fill-in*

Identify at least three goals for the management of patients in heart failure:

1. **Relieve patient symptoms**
2. **Improve functional status**
3. **Improve quality of life**
4. **Extend survival**

Exercise 1-31: *Calculation*

Order: Begin a dobutamine drip at 5 mcg/kg/min. James weighs 214 lb. The dobutamine is supplied as 500 mg in 250 mL of D5W.

Calculate how fast to run the dobutamine in mL/hr: **14.6 mL/hr.**

Exercise 1-32: *Fill-in*

Arterial blood gas (ABG) results:		
	pH	7.47
	pO_2	82
	pCO_2	30
	HCO_3	24

Evaluate the ABG above and explain why this is occurring.

Uncompensated respiratory alkalosis—James has labored breathing with a rate of 36 breaths/min; he is "blowing off" too much CO_2 resulting in a low pCO_2 and a higher than normal pH. The kidneys have not had time to compensate yet.

Exercise 1-33: *Matching*

Match the medication used to treat heart failure in Column A to its effect in Column B.

Column A		Column B
A. Benazepril	**D**	Beta blocker that reduces adverse effects from constant stimulation of the SNS
B. Furosemide	**E**	Catecholamine that increases cardiac contractility
C. Digoxin	**B**	Diuretic that removes excess extracellular fluid
D. Metoprolol	**F**	Phosphodiesterase inhibitor that promotes vasodilation
E. Dobutamine	**A**	ACE inhibitor that promotes vasodilation and diuresis
F. Milrinone	**C**	Cardiac glycoside that increases the force of myocardial contraction and slows conduction through the AV node

Exercise 1-34: *Multiple-choice question*

The nurse educating James on his medications for discharge determines that he needs further instruction about his diuretic when he states:

A. **"I can hold off taking my Lasix on days that I am traveling."—YES, Lasix should be taken as ordered and not held by the patient.**

B. "I should weigh myself every day at the same time."—NO, this is correct; it is best to weigh before breakfast.

C. "I should take my Lasix early in the day so I am not up all night."—NO

D. "I need to call the doctor if my legs start swelling more than normal."—NO, this may indicate that heart failure is worsening.

Exercise 1-35: *Select all that apply*

Since James will be discharged on digoxin, the nurse needs to discuss which of the following signs of digoxin toxicity?

☒ **Fatigue—YES**

☒ **Anorexia, nausea, vomiting—YES**

☒ **Changes in heart rate—YES, often the heart rate slows related to a block or the rhythm may become irregular indicating dysrhythmias.**

☒ **Changes in vision—YES, the patient may report a halo effect around objects or yellowed vision.**

Exercise 1-36: *Multiple-choice question*

After being connected to the heart monitor, the nurse identifies the following heart rhythm (Figure 1-4) as:

Figure 1-4: Cardiac Rhythm Strip

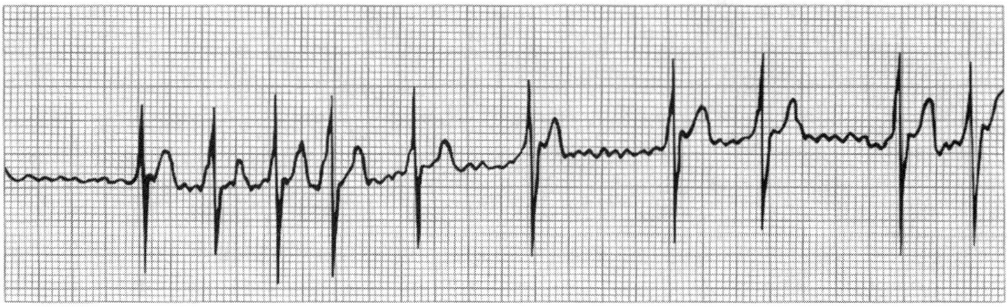

A. Sinus tachycardia—NO, this is a regular rhythm with P waves.

B. Atrial fibrillation—YES, this is an irregular rhythm with no discernible P wave.

C. Supraventricular tachycardia—NO, this is usually a regular rhythm.

D. Atrial flutter—NO, this is usually characterized by flutter waves.

Exercise 1-37: *Matching*

Match the ECG waves, complexes, or intervals in Column A to the electrical effects in the heart in Column B.

Column A	Column B
A. T wave	__E__ Early ventricular repolarization; isoelectric
B. PR interval	__C__ Ventricular depolarization
C. QRS complex	__D__ Atrial depolarization
D. P wave	__B__ Impulse travels from sinoatrial (SA) node
E. ST segment	through atrioventricular (AV) node
	__A__ Ventricular repolarization

Exercise 1-38: *Fill-in*

Identify common characteristics of atrial fibrillation:

1. Ventricular rate: **120–200 if untreated**

2. Ventricular and atrial rhythm: **Irregular**

3. P waves: **No discernible P waves; fibrillatory waves seen**

4. Q waves: **Usually normal**

5. P:QRS ratio: **Fibrillatory waves (no normal P wave): 1**

Exercise 1-39: *Calculation*

Order: Give a Cardizem bolus of 0.25 mg/kg. The patient weighs 190 pounds. Begin a Cardizem drip at 10 mg/hr. The Cardizem is supplied as 125 mg in 100 mL of D5W. Calculate the bolus to be given in mg: **21.6 mg**

Calculate how fast to run the Cardizem in mL/hr: **8 mL/hr.**

Exercise 1-40: *Select all that apply*

The nurse identifies that Marilyn has the following risk factors for developing atrial fibrillation:

☒ **Hypertension—YES**

☒ **Age—YES**

❏ Hypothyroidism—NO

☒ **Coronary artery disease—YES**

❏ Pulmonary disease—NO

Exercise 1-41: *Select all that apply*

Patients in atrial fibrillation exhibit signs and symptoms related to a rapid heart rate and the loss of AV synchrony. Identify common signs and symptoms of atrial fibrillation.

☒ **Irregular palpitations—YES**

❏ Nausea—NO

☒ **Shortness of breath—YES**

☒ **Fatigue—YES**

❏ Confusion—NO

Exercise 1-42: *Fill-in*

Explain how the low TSH level may be linked to the cause of the patient's atrial fibrillation.

When a patient is hyperthyroid, the TSH level will decline through a negative feedback mechanism. Marilyn has a history of hypothyroidism and has been taking the medication Synthroid. It is possible that her dose of Synthroid is too high, thus making her hyperthyroid and lowering TSH levels. Hyperthyroidism is one cause of atrial fibrillation.

Exercise 1-43: *Fill-in*

Patients in atrial fibrillation are often started on Coumadin because of the increased risk of: **an embolic event.**

Exercise 1-44: *Fill-in*

Identify the onset of action of Coumadin and the reason for this time frame.

Coumadin effects are seen in 36 to 72 hours after dosing begins. The reason for this delay is that Coumadin interferes with the new clotting factors being formed, but does not interfere with those already in circulation.

Exercise 1-45: *Fill-in*

In the event of overdose or excessive bleeding caused by Coumadin, the following antagonist can be given: **Vitamin K**

Exercise 1-46: *Select all that apply*

Identify the vitamin K-rich foods that can antagonize the effects of Coumadin:

☐ Potatoes—NO

☒ **Broccoli—YES**

☐ Oranges—NO

☒ **Green tea—YES**

☒ **Spinach—YES**

Exercise 1-47: *Multiple-choice question*

The nurse educating Marilyn on lab monitoring after discharge determines that she understands the instructions when she states:

A. "I only need to have my labs checked every 6 months."—NO, monitoring usually needs done more frequently, especially early in therapy.

B. "I have to have my PTT levels checked frequently."—NO, PTT levels are used to monitor the effects of heparin, not Coumadin.

C. "My INR level should be 0.8 to 1.2 while on Coumadin."—NO, this is the normal INR range for patients not taking anticoagulants.

D. **"I need to have my PT and INR levels drawn as instructed by my physician."—YES, the physician will prescribe how often these labs need to be drawn, taking into consideration dosage changes, side effects, and recent lab results.**

Exercise 1-48: *Multiple-choice question*

Identify the following heart rhythm (Figure 1-5):

Figure 1-5: Cardiac Rhythm Strip

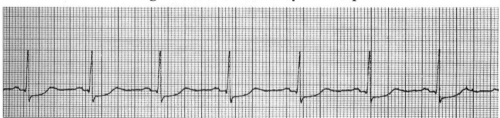

A. Junctional rhythm—NO, this is too fast for a junctional rhythm.

B. Atrial flutter—NO, there is no evidence of flutter waves.

C. **Sinus rhythm—YES, this is a normal rhythm.**

D. Sinus tachycardia—NO, this rhythm is not fast enough to be sinus tachycardia.

Exercise 1-49: *Fill-in*
Based upon the clinical manifestations that Barden is experiencing, the likely diagnosis is: **urinary tract infection with possible urosepsis.**

Exercise 1-50: *Fill-in*
Identify three signs or symptoms that suggest this diagnosis: **temperature 100.2°F, confusion**, and **urine is dark, cloudy with sediment, and foul smelling.**

Exercise 1-51: *Fill-in*
Identify whether the following abnormal laboratory results are elevated or decreased and why they are abnormal related to Barden's case.
1. White blood cells (WBCs) 23,000/cu mm **Elevated; WBCs increase with infection or inflammation; Barden has a urinary tract infection.**
2. Neutrophils 80% **Elevated; neutrophils increase with acute infections and are the primary defense against bacterial infections; Barden has a urinary tract infection.**
3. Lactic acid (venous) 22 mg/dL **Elevated; lactic acid increases in shock states; Barden has clinical manifestations of shock.**
4. pH 7.32 **Decreased; a pH less than 7.35 indicates acidosis, which can occur in shock states; Barden has clinical manifestations of shock.**
5. Creatinine 2.5 mg/dL **Elevated; creatinine elevates with dehydration and renal disease; Barden may be dehydrated, but he likely has some renal involvement as a result of his hypotension.**

Exercise 1-52: *Fill-in*
Antibiotics orders are written with the knowledge that, traditionally, the most common causative microorganism in septic shock is: **gram-negative bacteria**.

Exercise 1-53: *Matching*
Match the type of shock in Column A with its causative factors in Column B.

Column A		Column B
A. Hypovolemic	**C**	Loss of balance between parasympathetic and sympathetic stimulation
B. Cardiogenic	**D**	Widespread infection
C. Neurogenic	**A**	External fluid loss or internal fluid shifts
D. Septic	**E**	Severe allergic reaction
E. Anaphylactic	**B**	Stress or damage to the myocardium

Exercise 1-54: *Fill-in*

Identify the three stages of shock and associated clinical findings.

Stage 1: **Compensatory Stage**

     Blood pressure: **Normal**

     Heart rate: **> 100 bpm**

     Respirations: **> 20 breaths/min**

     Mentation: **Confused**

     Urine output: **Decreased**

Stage 2: **Progressive Stage**

     Blood pressure: **Systolic blood pressure < 80–90 mm Hg; requires fluids**

     Heart rate: **> 150 bpm**

     Respirations: **Rapid, shallow**

     Mentation: **Lethargic**

     Urine output: **Decreased**

Stage 3: **Irreversible Stage**

     Blood pressure: **Requires pharmacologic support**

     Heart rate: **Erratic; dysrhythmias common**

     Respirations: **Requires mechanical ventilation and oxygenation**

     Mentation: **Unconscious**

     Urine output: **Anuric (no urine output)**

Exercise 1-55: *Fill-in*

Based on the clinical manifestations that Barden is exhibiting, he is likely in the **progressive** stage of shock.

Exercise 1-56: *Multiple-choice question*

When discussing urosepsis and septic shock with her orientee, the nurse identifies which common clinical manifestations?

A. Hypotension, tachycardia, and metabolic alkalosis—NO, metabolic alkalosis is incorrect; the patient is acidotic.

B. Cool/clammy skin, bradycardia, and metabolic alkalosis—NO, bradycardia and metabolic alkalosis are incorrect; the patient is tachycardic.

C. Normal respirations, hypotension, and cool/clammy skin—NO, respirations are not normal, but rather rapid and shallow or requiring ventilatory support.

D. Tachycardia, decreased urine output, and metabolic acidosis—YES, these are all characteristic of the shock state.

Exercise 1-57: *Select all that apply*

Identify therapies used in the treatment of septic shock:

☒ **Fluid replacement—YES**

☐ Progressive activity—NO

☒ **Vasoactive drugs—YES**

☒ **Nutritional support—YES**

☒ **Early antibiotics—YES**

❑ Aggressive hypothermia—NO

Exercise 1-58: *Calculation*

Order: Begin a Levophed drip at 2 mcg/min. The Levophed is supplied as 4 mg in 500 mL of D5W.

Calculate how fast to run the Levophed in mL/hr: **15 mL/hr**

Exercise 1-59: *Multiple-choice question*

In dealing with patients and families who are facing critical illness and potential death, it is important for the nurse to:

  A. Reassure the patient and family that everything will be okay—NO, never give false reassurance.

  B. Maintain a strict visitation schedule—NO, advocate for family presence when appropriate.

  C. **Speak in a calm, reassuring voice using touch as appropriate—YES, this may provide comfort and ease patient and family concerns.**

  D. Provide long, detailed explanations—NO, explanations should be brief.

Exercise 1-60: *Fill-in*

Taking into account Marcey's current complaint and her past medical history, the nurse determines that Marcey is likely experiencing **intermittent claudication** related to **peripheral arterial insufficiency**.

Exercise 1-61: *Select all that apply*

Identify physical assessment changes that can be seen as a result of inadequate arterial blood flow to the extremities:

☒ **Loss of hair—YES**

☒ **Decreased or absent pulses—YES**

❑ Severe edema—NO, more commonly seen with venous disorders.

☒ **Cool, pale skin—YES**

❑ Ulcers near the medial malleolus—NO, more commonly seen with venous disorders.

☒ **Rubor when extremities are dependent—YES**

Exercise 1-62: *Calculation*

Calculate the ABI for each foot by dividing the highest ankle systolic pressure by the higher of the two brachial systolic pressures.

Right ABI = **90/140 mm Hg = 0.64**

Left ABI = **80/140 mm Hg = 0.57**

Exercise 1-63: *Select all that apply*
Identify the modifiable risk factors associated with peripheral arterial disease:
❑ Age—NO, this is a nonmodifiable risk factor.
☒ **Nicotine use—YES**
❑ Familial predisposition—NO, this is a nonmodifiable risk factor.
☒ **Sedentary lifestyle—YES**
☒ **Hypertension—YES**
☒ **Stress—YES**

Exercise 1-64: *Fill-in*
Marcey has several risk factors for peripheral arterial disease that further increase her risk of future heart disease. Identify those risk factors that are modifiable. **Nicotine use**, **hypertension**, **dyslipidemia**, and **obesity**.

Exercise 1-65: *Multiple-choice question*
The nurse educating Marcey on risk factor modification determines that she understands the instructions when she states:
A. "I have been smoking a long time, but I will try to cut back some."—NO, she needs to quit smoking altogether to minimize her risk.
B. **"I need to alter my diet to reduce my calories, fat, and cholesterol intake."—YES, weight loss and controlling her dyslipidemia are important to modify her risk.**
C. "If I change my diet, I can stop taking my cholesterol medication."—NO, she should not stop any medication unless instructed to do so by her physician.
D. "I need to cut back on my activity and avoid all exercise."—NO, a sedentary lifestyle is a risk factor; activity and exercise will assist with weight loss; rest when pain occurs.

Exercise 1-66: *True or false*
Identify whether the following statements are true or false:
__True__ 1. People with peripheral arterial insufficiency should position the affected extremity below the level of the heart to improve circulation.
__True__ 2. Elevating the head of the bed on 6-inch blocks will improve arterial circulation.
__False__ 3. People with peripheral arterial insufficiency should continue exercising even with pain in the affected extremity.

Exercise 1-67: *Select all that apply*
Identify interventions effective in promoting vasodilation and/or preventing compression:
☒ **Avoid cold temperatures—YES, cold causes vasoconstriction.**
❑ Use heating pads or hot water bottles on affected extremities—NO

☒ Avoid crossing legs—YES, this may impede circulation to the extremities.

☒ Avoid tight clothing—YES, this may impede circulation to the extremities.

☒ Encourage stress management—YES, stress stimulates the sympathetic nervous system, causing vasoconstriction.

Exercise 1-68: *Fill-in*

Briefly explain how nicotine negatively affects people with peripheral arterial disease. **Nicotine causes vasospasm, which reduces circulation to the extremities. Tobacco smoke also impairs the transport and use of oxygen at the cellular level.**

Exercise 1-69: *Multiple-choice question*

The nurse educating Marcey on methods for protecting her extremities determines that she needs further instruction when she states:

A. "I should check my feet every day and notify my physician of any problems."—NO

B. "When my feet get dry and scaly, I rub them with a hard-bristled brush."— YES, this may interrupt skin integrity and increase the risk of infection.

C. "I should wear well-fitting shoes or slippers at all times."—NO

D. "I should avoid using lotion between my toes."—NO

Exercise 1-70: *Fill-in*

Identify at least four complications that can occur with an arteriogram: **allergic reaction to the contrast dye, blood clot at the catheter insertion site, blood clot that travels to the lungs, damage to the blood vessel, excessive bleeding at the catheter insertion site, heart attack or stroke, hematoma at the catheter insertion site, nerve injury, or kidney damage from the dye.**

Exercise 1-71: *Select all that apply*

Identify the nursing interventions appropriate for the care of a patient post angiogram:

☒ **Assess peripheral pulses in the affected extremity beginning at every 15 minutes—YES**

☒ **Monitor the insertion site for bleeding or hematoma—YES**

❑ Keep head of bed higher than 30 degrees—NO, keep head of bed lower than 30 degrees.

❑ Limit oral fluid intake—NO, encourage fluid intake to flush dye from the kidneys.

☒ **Assess temperature and color of affected extremity—YES**

Exercise 1-72: *Fill-in*

After completing her assessment and reviewing Margaret's chief complaint and past medical/surgical history, the nurse suspects that she has: **deep vein thrombosis.**

Exercise 1-73: *Fill-in*

Virchow's triad is believed to play a significant role in the development of venous thromboembolism (VTE). List the three factors that comprise Virchow's triad:

1. **Venous stasis**
2. **Vessel wall injury**
3. **Altered blood coagulation**

Exercise 1-74: *Fill-in*

Briefly identify Margaret's risk factors for developing deep vein thrombosis and then connect them with the factors of Virchow's triad.

1. **67 years old; there is increased risk of venous stasis associated with ages greater than 65 years.**
2. **Obesity; there is increased risk of venous stasis associated with obesity.**
3. **Recent right knee replacement; there is increased risk of vessel wall injury associated with surgery.**
4. **Decreased mobility postoperatively; there is increased risk of venous stasis associated with bed rest and immobilization.**

Exercise 1-75: *Select all that apply*

Identify which laboratory tests must be checked prior to beginning Lovenox and then monitored during the course of therapy:

☒ **Platelets—YES, this is done to monitor for thrombocytopenia.**

❑ Potassium—NO

❑ D-dimer—NO

☒ **Hemoglobin/hematocrit—YES, this is done to detect bleeding that may occur while on anticoagulant therapy.**

☒ **aPTT—YES, this is done prior to starting therapy to check for an existing coagulation problem; it may be checked intermittently during therapy with certain populations (patients who are obese or have renal insufficiency).**

Exercise 1-76: *Select all that apply*

Identify clinical manifestations associated with deep vein thrombosis:

☒ **Warmth in the calf area—YES, the affected leg may feel warmer.**

☒ **Edema—YES, venous outflow is inhibited.**

☒ **Functional impairment—YES, may occur related to swelling and pain.**

❑ Absence of dorsalis pedis pulse—NO, arterial blood flow is not affected.

☒ **Differences in leg circumference bilaterally—YES, swelling enlarges the affected leg.**

Exercise 1-77: *Fill-in*

Briefly explain how Homans' sign is performed and how it is used to assess for deep vein thrombosis: **A patient has a positive Homans' sign when he or she experiences pain in the calf as the foot is sharply dorsiflexed. Homans' sign is not a reliable indicator for deep vein thrombosis because it can occur with any painful condition of the leg.**

Exercise 1-78: *True or false*

Identify whether the following statements about prevention of deep vein thrombosis are true or false:

  False 1. Antiembolism stockings are ineffective in preventing deep vein thrombosis.

  True 2. Early mobilization after surgery is an effective prevention therapy.

  True 3. Low-molecular-weight heparin is an effective prophylaxis used after certain surgeries.

Exercise 1-79: *Calculation*

Order: Give enoxaparin (Lovenox) 1 mg/kg subcutaneously every 12 hours. The patient's weight is 197 pounds.

Calculate the dose of Lovenox to be given in mg: **90 mg**

Exercise 1-80: *Multiple-choice question*

The nurse educating Margaret on the action of Lovenox determines that she understands the information when she states that Lovenox will:

A. "Dissolve the clot in my leg and prevent new ones from forming."—NO, Lovenox does not dissolve existing thrombi.

B. **"Prevent the clot in my leg from getting bigger and prevent new ones from forming."—YES, Lovenox can only prevent extension of existing thrombi and formation of new ones.**

C. "Prevent the clot in my leg from getting bigger and eventually dissolve it."—NO, Lovenox does not dissolve existing thrombi.

D. "Cause the clot in my leg to move and break apart."—NO, Lovenox does not cause thrombi to move; a thrombus breaking loose could result in pulmonary emboli.

Exercise 1-81: *Hot spot*
Mark the areas (Figure 1-6) where you would administer the Lovenox:

Figure 1-6: Abdomen

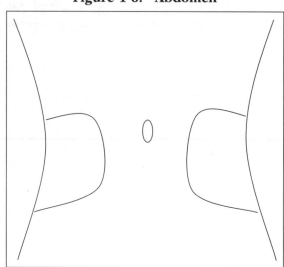

Exercise 1-82: *Multiple-choice question*
The nurse educating Margaret on her medications for discharge determines that she needs further instruction about Lovenox when she states:
A. "I should notify the physician if I see any blood in my urine."—NO
B. "I should avoid giving my Lovenox in the same location every day."—NO
C. "I am at increased risk for bleeding while on Lovenox and Coumadin."—NO
D. "I have to have my aPTT monitored every day while on Lovenox."—YES, aPTT does not need to be monitored daily while on Lovenox; this is required with intravenous unfractionated heparin.

Exercise 1-83: *Select all that apply*
Since Margaret has been on anticoagulants for 3 days, what activities would you recommend that she continue at home?
☒ **Elevate her right leg when recumbent—YES, this helps reduce swelling.**
☐ Begin walking on a treadmill as soon as possible—NO, this could be dangerous.
☒ **Progressively increase her ambulation—YES, this prevents further problems associated with immobility.**
☒ **Repetitively dorsiflex both feet when recumbent—YES, this increases venous return.**
☐ Keep her knees bent when sitting in the recliner—NO, this increases the risk of clot development.

Exercise 1-84: *Matching*

Match the arterial or venous insufficiency in Column A with its typical characteristics in Column B. Answers in Column A can be used more than once.

<table>
<tr><th>Column A</th><th colspan="2">Column B</th></tr>
<tr><td>A. Arterial insufficiency</td><td>__**B**__</td><td>Aching, cramping type pain</td></tr>
<tr><td>B. Venous insufficiency</td><td>__**B**__</td><td>Skin thickened, tough, and pigmented</td></tr>
<tr><td></td><td>__**A**__</td><td>Pulses diminished or absent</td></tr>
<tr><td></td><td>__**B**__</td><td>Edema moderate to severe</td></tr>
<tr><td></td><td>__**A**__</td><td>Ulcers usually on tips of toes or heels</td></tr>
<tr><td></td><td>__**A**__</td><td>Often very painful</td></tr>
</table>

2

Nursing Care of the Patient
With Pulmonary Disease

Rhonda M. Brogdon

Unfolding Case Study #8 ■ Victor

Victor is a 56-year-old patient who received a cholecystectomy when admitted to the hospital. He is now 3 days postoperation and on the surgical unit. Upon morning assessment, the nurse auscultated diminished lung sounds anteriorly in the right lung base and the patient complained of a cough. Victor's vital signs are: blood pressure 138/89, pulse 126, respirations 26, temperature 101.1°F, and an oxygen saturation of 88%.

Exercise 2-1: *Fill-in*
The nurse suspects the diagnosis of _____.

The primary care provider has ordered a STAT chest x-ray, complete blood count (CBC), a basic metabolic panel (BMP), arterial blood gases (ABGs), and oxygen at 2 L/min per nasal cannula.

Exercise 2-2: *Fill-in*
Arterial blood gas results reveal a pH of 7.30, PCO_2 of 55, and HCO_3 of 26. What is this blood gas interpretation? _____

e **eResource 2-1:** Use MedCalc's Acid–Base Online Calculator to verify your understanding: [Pathway: www.medcalc.com → select "Pulmonary" → select "ABG Calculator" and enter patient data]

Exercise 2-3: *Select all that apply*
The nurse identifies the following risk factors or manifestations of atelectasis:

- ❏ Abdominal surgery
- ❏ Decreased or absent breath sounds
- ❏ Equal chest movement
- ❏ Rapid heart rate
- ❏ Fever
- ❏ Confinement to bed

Answers to this chapter begin on page 67.

The nurse completed Victor's physical assessment. Victor has been confined to bed for 3 days because of his complaint of unrelieved pain. The nurse knows that Victor's manifestations require immediate intervention.

Exercise 2-4: *Fill-in*

Victor's clinical manifestations require immediate intervention and assessment by the primary care provider. Identify at least three of Victor's clinical manifestations: _____, _____, and _____.

Exercise 2-5: *Fill-in*

The nurse informs Victor that his physical assessment findings require immediate testing to conclude atelectasis. What three ways can you diagnose atelectasis?

1. _____

2. _____

3. _____

e **eResource 2-2:** To learn more about atelectasis and its diagnosis, visit Medscape:
- Online: [Pathway: www.medscape.org → Under the tab "Reference," select "References & Tools" → enter "atelectasis" into the search field → review "Presentation," "DDx" and "Workup"]
- On your mobile device: [Pathway: Medscape → enter "atelectasis" into the search field → review "Presentation," "DDx" and "Workup"]

After Victor was assessed by the primary care provider (PCP), the nurse reviews the plan of care and treatment regimen with Victor, which includes: (a) physical therapy, (b) respiratory therapy, and (c) medications.

Exercise 2-6: *Select all that apply*

When educating patients about atelectasis, the nurse includes the following information:
- ❑ Turn, cough, and deep breathe
- ❑ Incentive spirometry
- ❑ Chest percussion and postural drainage
- ❑ Assess breath sounds every 12 hours

e **eResource 2-3:** To supplement patient teaching, the nurse shows Victor a video tutorial, *Atelectasis*: http://youtu.be/FhFpbZcIIzQ

Victor is instructed on the use of incentive spirometry.

Exercise 2-7: *Multiple-choice question*

The nurse understands that Victor needs further teaching in the use of incentive spirometry when he states:
- A. "I only have to use it when I can't breathe."
- B. "I am to use it every hour for 10 to 20 breaths while awake."

C. "I can continue to use it once I go home to keep my lungs clear."

D. "I am to hold the incentive spirometer in an upright position."

 eResource 2-4: The nurse shows Victor a video demonstrating the use of the incentive spirometer: http://youtu.be/cWBj5o5NblY

In addition to incentive spirometry, medications can also be used to treat Victor's atelectasis.

Exercise 2-8: *Fill-in*

Name three medications that can be used to treat atelectasis:

_____, _____, and _____.

Unfolding Case Study #9 ▨ William

William is a 67-year-old patient who has come to the emergency department (ED) complaining of a low-grade fever of 99.5°F, a productive cough of yellow mucus, chills, weakness, and shortness of breath with activities. When assessing William's lungs, the nurse auscultated crackles in the right middle lobe and left upper lobe anteriorly.

 eResource 2-5: To hear samples of lung sounds, go to:
- *Crackles—Early Inspiratory (Rales):* http://goo.gl/gUx17
- *Crackles—Fine (Rales):* http://goo.gl/vBr2h
- *Crackles—Coarse (Rales):* http://goo.gl/e2FR1

Exercise 2-9: *Fill-in*

Based on the patient's symptoms, the nurse suspects William may have

_____.

Exercise 2-10: *Select all that apply*

The most common symptoms of pneumonia are:

❑ Cough

❑ Fever

❑ Shaking chills

❑ Shortness of breath

❑ Weakness/fatigue

❑ Excessive sweating

❑ Increased appetite

Answers to this chapter begin on page 67.

Exercise 2-11: *Select all that apply*

Based on William's symptoms, what can lead to his greatest risk for pneumonia?

❏ Older than 65

❏ Cigarette smoking

❏ Asthma

❏ Recent cold or flu

❏ Pneumococcal vaccine every 5 years

eResource 2-6: To learn more about risk for pneumonia, consult the Pneumonia Severity Index Calculator: http://goo.gl/CgxSN

The nurse has completed the physical assessment and health history on William. William has a history of pneumonia, was a smoker for 10 years, and has asthma. After being assessed by the primary care provider (PCP), William is scheduled for a chest x-ray, a CBC, blood cultures times two prior to antibiotics, ABGs, and a sputum culture. The PCP has ordered for the patient to receive Levaquin 750 mg by mouth after the scheduled tests are completed.

eResource 2-7: To verify that this is the correct dosage, consult Skyscape's RxDrugs on your mobile device: [Pathway: RxDrugs → enter "levaquin" into the search field and check adult dosing]

The nurse completes Levaquin education with William.

Exercise 2-12: *Fill-in*

Identify at least three potential adverse effects of Levaquin:

1. _____

2. _____

3. _____

Exercise 2-13: *Select all that apply*

After further education about Levaquin, the nurse asks William what medications he should be cautious of while taking Levaquin:

❏ Antacids

❏ Magnesium

❏ Iron

❏ Zinc

❏ Potassium

❏ Albuterol

Answers to this chapter begin on page 67.

eResource 2-8: Consult Epocrates to learn/review safety and monitoring guidelines related to Levaquin: [Pathway: Epocrates → select "Levaquin" → select "Safety/Monitoring." Also review Contraindications/Cautions as well as Adverse Reactions for further patient teaching]

Exercise 2-14: *Multiple-choice question*
After education about Levaquin, the nurse determines that William needs further instruction when he states:

    A. "I will not drive until I know how this medication will affect me."

    B. "I will stay out of the sun or use sunscreen."

    C. "I will take my Zantac at the same time as my Levaquin."

    D. "If I have changes in my vision, I will notify my doctor."

Unfolding Case Study #10 ▨ Caleb

Caleb is a 28-year-old patient who presents to the emergency department (ED) with dyspnea and audible wheezing. The nurse assessed a productive cough, fever of 101.5°F, tachypnea at 32 breaths/min, and tachycardia at 118 beats/min. His pulse oximetry is 88% on room air.

 eResource 2-9: To learn more about respiratory wheezing, listen to the Merck Manual of Patient Symptoms Podcast, *Wheezing*: http://goo.gl/BA2cb

Exercise 2-15: *Fill-in*
Based on Caleb's physical assessment, he is exhibiting clinical manifestations of:
_____.

 eResource 2-10: To hear other samples of wheezing lung sounds, go to:
▪ *Wheeze*: http://goo.gl/692Fm
▪ *Wheezes—Expiratory*: http://goo.gl/azJjo
▪ *Wheezes—Monophonic*: http://goo.gl/P64fE
▪ *Wheezes—Polyphonic*: http://goo.gl/G3PDI

Exercise 2-16: *Fill-in*
The primary care provider has assessed Caleb and has ordered ABGs, chest x-ray, pulmonary function tests, and a sputum culture. Caleb's medical history includes smoker for 4 years, and a recent admission for asthma 3 weeks ago. Which test is the most accurate for diagnosing asthma and its severity? _____

 eResource 2-11: Consult Epocrates Online to review content related to prevention of asthma: [Pathway: https://online.epocrates.com → under the "Diseases" tab, enter "asthma" in the search field → select "Asthma in adults" Under "Diagnosis" select "Approach"]

Answers to this chapter begin on page 67.

Exercise 2-17: *Select all that apply*
Which of Caleb's manifestations indicate a deterioration in his respiratory status?
- ❏ Arterial oxygen saturation (SaO_2) of 88%
- ❏ Audible wheezing
- ❏ Tachypnea at 32 breaths/min
- ❏ Tachycardia at 118 beats/min
- ❏ Age of 28

Exercise 2-18: *Fill-in*
Based on Caleb's manifestations, the nurse can expect to administer what classification of medication for his acute symptoms? _____

Exercise 2-19: *Fill-in*
Identify three adverse effects of bronchodilators.

1. _____
2. _____
3. _____

Exercise 2-20: *Fill-in*
After administering medication education to Caleb, name three nursing considerations that should be monitored.

1. _____
2. _____
3. _____

eResource 2-12: To learn more about bronchodilators, go to Epocrates Online to review content related to prevention: [Pathway: https://online.epocrates.com → under the "Diseases" tab, enter "asthma" in the search field → select "Asthma in adults" Under "Diagnosis" select "Approach"]

Exercise 2-21: *Select all that apply*
Potential irritants of asthma include:
- ❏ House dust mites
- ❏ Mold or yeast spores
- ❏ Cat hair and saliva
- ❏ Cockroach particles
- ❏ Smoke
- ❏ Exercise

Answers to this chapter begin on page 67.

eResource 2-13: To learn more about asthma and its triggers, visit Medscape:
- Online: [Pathway: www.medscape.org → Under the tab "Reference," select "References & Tools" → enter "asthma" into the search field → under the "Overview" tab, review "Pathophysiology" and "Etiology"]
- On your mobile device, you can access the same information: [Pathway: Medscape → enter "asthma" into the search field → under the "Overview" tab, review "Pathophysiology" and "Etiology"]

Exercise 2-22: *Select all that apply*

Clinical manifestations of asthma include:

- ❑ Increased respiratory rate
- ❑ Wheezing
- ❑ Productive cough
- ❑ Use of accessory muscles
- ❑ Dyspnea
- ❑ Dry skin

 eResource 2-14: To reinforce patient teaching, the nurse plays the CDC podcast, *Asthma—What You Need to Know:* http://goo.gl/KCpa8

Exercise 2-23: *Exhibit question*

Caleb's ABG result is as follows:

pH = 7.21
PO_2 = 66
PCO_2 = 55
HCO_3 = 22

Evaluate the ABG result above and explain why it is occurring.

_____

_____

_____

 eResource 2-15: Use MedCalc's Acid–Base Online Calculator to verify your understanding: [Pathway: www.medcalc.com → select "Pulmonary" → select "ABG Calculator" and enter patient data]

Caleb's condition has improved after his dosing of medications.

Exercise 2-24: *Matching*
Match the medication used to treat asthma in Column A to its effect in Column B.

Column A	Column B
A. Ventolin	_____ Increases contraction of the diaphragm
B. Atrovent	_____ Decreases airway inflammation
C. Theo-dur	_____ Rapid relief of acute symptoms
D. Prednisone	_____ Blocks the parasympathetic nervous system

Exercise 2-25: *Select all that apply*
Upon discharge from the emergency department, the nurse explains to Caleb that it is important that he maintains good health. Some positive patient outcomes for Caleb would include:

❑ Decreases exposure to irritants

❑ Identifies mechanisms for coping

❑ Maintains adequate respiratory function

❑ Not getting his family involved in his care

Exercise 2-26: *Fill-in*
Caleb is taught the importance of health promotion and disease prevention with asthma. What are three ways that can help Caleb improve his quality of life with asthma?

1. _____

2. _____

3. _____

 eResource 2-16: To help Caleb understand what he can do to manage his asthma, the nurse shows him a video, *Living With and Managing Asthma:* http://youtu.be/ImYZd6KxO8c

Unfolding Case Study #11 ▬ Joshua

Joshua is a 49-year-old patient who has been diagnosed with chronic obstructive pulmonary disease (COPD). He has episodic dyspnea and purulent sputum production. His physical assessment by the nurse reveals expiratory wheezes and inspiratory rhonchi in the right lung base and clubbing of his fingernails. Joshua's blood pressure is 138/80, pulse 100, respiratory rate of 22, oxygen saturation of 85%, and a temperature of 99.0°F. His medical history includes smoking three packs of cigarettes a day, and presently he smokes one pack a day.

Exercise 2-27: *Fill-in*

Identify four causes of COPD.

1. _____

2. _____

3. _____

4. _____

eResource 2-17: To learn more about COPD and its diagnosis, visit Medscape:
- Online: [Pathway: www.medscape.org → Under the tab "Reference," select "References & Tools" → enter "COPD" into the search field → Under "Overview," select "etiology"]
- On your mobile device: [Pathway: Medscape → enter "COPD" into the search field → Under "Overview," select "etiology"]

The primary care provider (PCP) has examined Joshua and has ordered a CBC, oxygen at 2 L/min, pulse oximetry, ABGs, sputum culture, pulmonary function tests, chest x-ray, and medication management.

Exercise 2-28: *Calculation*

Calculate aminophylline intravenous (IV) loading dose of 5 mg/kg over 30 minutes followed by 0.5 mg/kg/hr continuous IV. Calculate mL/hr to set the IV pump for the loading dose of aminophylline for Joshua who weighs 160 pounds. The aminophylline supply is 100 mg/100 mL D5W.

_____

_____

_____

Exercise 2-29: *Calculation*

Calculate mL/hr to set the IV pump for the continuous dose of aminophylline for Joshua. The aminophylline is supplied as 1 g/250 mL D5W.

_____

_____

eResource 2-18: Use MedCalc to verify your answer: [Pathway: www.medcalc.com → select "Fluids/Electrolytes" → select "IV Rate" and enter information into fields]

Exercise 2-30: *Fill-in*

What is the consideration of oxygen therapy in COPD patients?

_____

_____

Answers to this chapter begin on page 67.

e **eResource 2-19:** To learn more about oxygen therapy for a patient with COPD, view *Administering Oxygen in COPD*: http://youtu.be/6h0Ea4Tc-Qk

Exercise 2-31: *Multiple-choice question*
Joshua's ABG results revealed a pH of 7.30, PaO_2 of 50, PCO_2 of 48, and a HCO_3 of 26. What is Joshua's ABG interpretation?

    A. Metabolic alkalosis
    B. Respiratory acidosis
    C. Metabolic acidosis
    D. Respiratory alkalosis

e **eResource 2-20:** Use MedCalc's Acid–Base Online Calculator to verify your understanding: [Pathway: www.medcalc.com → select "Pulmonary" → select "ABG Calculator" and enter patient data]

e **eResource 2-21:** To learn more about COPD and its diagnosis, visit Medscape:
    ■ Online: [Pathway: www.medscape.org → Under the tab "Reference," select "References & Tools" → enter "COPD" into the search field → Under "Treatment," select "Oxygen Therapy and Hypoxemia"]
    ■ On your mobile device: [Pathway: Medscape → enter "COPD" into the search field → Under "Treatment," select "Oxygen Therapy and Hypoxemia"]

Exercise 2-32: *Fill-in*
What classification of medications will be administered to Joshua to relieve his symptoms?

    1. _____
    2. _____
    3. _____
    4. _____

Exercise 2-33: *Fill-in*
Identify two types of breathing techniques to control Joshua's dyspneic episodes.

    1. _____
    2. _____

e **eResource 2-22:** To learn more about breathing techniques for a patient with COPD, view *Managing an Episode of Acute Shortness of Breath*: http://youtu.be/wUr0YVZuM5M

Answers to this chapter begin on page 67.

Exercise 2-34: *Fill-in*

Incentive spirometry is used to monitor Joshua's lung expansion. What education is given to the patient regarding how to use the incentive spirometry?

_____

_____

e **eResource 2-23:** To learn more about the proper technique for using incentive spirometry, view http://youtu.be/VHN5zPaw96w

Exercise 2-35: *Select all that apply*

The nurse knows that promoting adequate nutrition is important while Joshua is in the hospital. What education is given to Joshua on the importance of nutrition?

❑ Encourage 2 to 3 L/day of fluid

❑ How to prevent infection

❑ High-calorie and high-protein diet

❑ Consume caffeine

❑ Avoid caffeine

Exercise 2-36: *Fill-in*

While in the hospital, other interdisciplinary care teams have been consulted for Joshua. What is the importance of respiratory services, nutritional services, and rehabilitative care?

Respiratory services: _____

Nutritional services: _____

Rehabilitative services: _____

Exercise 2-37: *Select all that apply*

Upon discharge from the hospital, what education is given to Joshua to improve his quality of care since his diagnosis of COPD?

❑ Encourage smoking cessation

❑ Encourage influenza and pneumonia vaccines

❑ Promote hand hygiene to prevent infection

❑ Discontinue medications once feeling better

❑ Report fluid retention and weight gain

e **eResource 2-24:** Consult Epocrates Online for detailed information related to discharge teaching and follow-up for Joshua: [Pathway: https://online.epocrates.com → select "Diseases" → enter "COPD" in the search field → select "Follow-Up" and review content]

Answers to this chapter begin on page 67.

Unfolding Case Study #12 ▦ Patterson

Patterson is a 30-year-old patient who is being admitted into the hospital for overnight observation. She has a complaint of dyspnea (shortness of breath), a productive cough, and pain along with erythema and tenderness in her right lower leg. Patterson has a history of smoking illegal substances (marijuana) and smoking three packs of cigarettes a day; she is currently using estrogen for irregular menstrual cycles and now smokes one pack of cigarettes a day. Her blood pressure is 128/88, respiratory rate of 22, pulse 110, oxygen saturation of 90%, and temperature of 99.5°F.

Exercise 2-38: *Fill-in*
The nurse suspects Patterson of having a _____.

Exercise 2-39: *Select all that apply*
Risk factors associated with pulmonary embolism include:

❑ Pregnancy

❑ Tobacco use

❑ Oral contraceptive and estrogen therapy

❑ Decreased platelet count

❑ Long-term immobility

The primary care provider (PCP) has ordered a chest x-ray and/or a computed tomographic (CT) scan of the chest, ventilation and perfusion scan (V/Q scan), D-dimer, CBC, and ABGs.

Exercise 2-40: *Fill-in*
What is the significance in ordering a chest x-ray and a V/Q scan?

_____

_____

e **eResource 2-25:** To learn more about this procedure, consult the Merck Manual: [Pathway: www.merckmanuals.com → select "The Merck Manual of Diagnosis and Therapy" → enter "ventilation and perfusion scan" into the search field in the upper right corner → select "V/Q scanning" and review content]

The nurse reported the D-dimer results to the PCP. The results indicated a positive D-dimer of 4.0 mcg/mL. The expected reference range is 0.43 to 2.33 mcg/mL.

Exercise 2-41: *Fill-in*
What does the positive D-dimer signify to the nurse and the primary care provider?

_____

_____

Answers to this chapter begin on page 67.

eResource 2-26: Consult Epocrates Online for detailed information regarding diagnostic tests for pulmonary embolism: [Pathway: https://online.epocrates.com → select "Diseases" → enter "pulmonary embolisim" in the search field → select "Diagnosis" → select "Tests" and review content. Be sure to click on "D-dimer" to view detailed information]

The nurse knows that Patterson has been diagnosed with a pulmonary embolism according to the diagnostic testing.

Exercise 2-42: *Fill-in*

What three types of medications can be administered for pulmonary embolism?

1. _____

2. _____

3. _____

The PCP has ordered heparin 5000 units IV push followed by a continuous IV infusion of 1000 units/hr.

Exercise 2-43: *Calculation*

Calculate how many mL of heparin bolus Patterson will receive IV from a multidose vial labeled 10,000 units/mL.

_____

_____

Calculate mL/hr to set the IV pump for the continuous dose of heparin. Heparin is supplied as 25,000 units/250 mL D5W.

_____

_____

 eResource 2-27: Use MedCalc to verify your calculations:
- Online: [Pathway: www.medcalc.com → select "Fluids/Electrolytes" → select "IV Rate" and enter infusion order]
- Mobile device: [Pathway: MedCalc → enter "infusion" into the search field → select "Infusion Management" → enter infusion order]

Exercise 2-44: *Select all that apply*

What type of education is given to Patterson in the treatment and prevention of a pulmonary embolism?

❑ Promote smoking cessation

❑ Encourage wearing of compression stockings to promote circulation

❑ Avoid crossing legs

❑ Avoid long periods of immobility

❑ Discourage physical activity such as walking

Answers to this chapter begin on page 67.

Exercise 2-45: *Fill-in*
Upon discharge from the hospital, the nurse should instruct Patterson on increased risk for bruising and bleeding while on anticoagulants. What should Patterson know?

_____

_____

_____

 eResource 2-28: To supplement the patient teaching regarding anticoagulant therapy, visit Medscape:
- Online: [Pathway: www.medscape.org → Under the tab "Reference," select "References & Tools" → enter "Pulmonary Embolism" into the search field → under "Medication," select "Anticoagulants"]
- On your mobile device: [Pathway: Medscape → "Pulmonary Embolism" into the search field → Under "Medication," select "Anticoagulants"]

Exercise 2-46: *Multiple-choice question*
After discharge education has been completed, the nurse knows that Patterson needs further instructions when she states:
- A. "I will adhere to anticoagulant therapy."
- B. "I will wear my compression stockings to promote circulation."
- C. "I will only smoke three times a week."
- D. "I will check my mouth and skin daily for bleeding and bruising."

 eResource 2-29: For more information regarding patient teaching, consult Epocrates Online: [Pathway: https://online.epocrates.com → select "Diseases" → enter "pulmonary embolisim" in the search field → select "Follow-up" → select "Overview" and review content. Be sure to view "Prevention" to learn about secondary prevention measures]

Unfolding Case Study #13 ▪ Martha

Martha is a 56-year-old patient who presents to the emergency department (ED) complaining of episodes of dyspnea (shortness of breath). She has a past medical history of a myocardial infarction, hypertension, and left-sided heart failure. The nurse auscultated inspiratory crackles, blood pressure of 148/96, tachycardia of 120 beats/min, tachypnea of 28 breaths/min, and a productive cough of pink frothy sputum. Martha's skin is pale in color and cool to touch. Martha stated that she has had a recent "weight gain of 20 pounds and has swollen ankles and feet."

 eResource 2-30: To hear how inspiratory crackles sound, go to: http://goo.gl/gUx17

Exercise 2-47: *Fill-in*

What does the nurse suspect Martha's subjective and objective data results mean she has?

_____

Exercise 2-48: *Fill-in*

Identify three of Martha's risk factors for pulmonary edema.

1. _____

2. _____

3. _____

> **eResource 2-31:** For more information regarding risk factors for pulmonary edema, consult Epocrates Online: [Pathway: https://online .epocrates.com → select "Diseases" → enter "pulmonary edema" in the search field → under "Diagnosis" select "Risk Factors"]

The primary care provider (PCP) has admitted Martha into the hospital after his assessment. The PCP has ordered a chest x-ray, ABGs, and diuretics.

Exercise 2-49: *Fill-in*

The primary care provider has ordered two diuretics, furosemide (Lasix) and bumetanide (Bumex), to alleviate fluid overload. What does the nurse know about these medications?

_____

_____

> **eResource 2-32:** To learn more about these drugs and precautions, consult Skyscape's RxDrugs on your mobile device: [Pathway: Skyscape → select "RxDrugs" → enter "Lasix" into the search field → scroll down to view Warnings/precautions; repeat with "Bumex"]

> **eResource 2-33:** To learn more about the action of diuretics in the kidney, view: http://youtu.be/6Wc4f2KnbYo

Exercise 2-50: *Select all that apply*

What type of nursing care is imperative for Martha in order to achieve positive health outcomes?

❏ Monitor intake and output

❏ Maintain intravenous fluids

❏ Maintain a patent airway

❏ Restrict fluid intake

❏ Monitor hourly urine output

Answers to this chapter begin on page 67.

Exercise 2-51: *Fill-in*

Upon discharge, the nurse will educate Martha on the importance of health promotion and disease prevention for pulmonary edema. What type of information can be taught?

_____

_____

_____

 eResource 2-34: For more information regarding risk factors for pulmonary edema, consult Epocrates Online: [Pathway: https://online .epocrates.com → select "Diseases" → enter "pulmonary edema" in the search field → under "Follow-up" select "Patient Teaching"]

Unfolding Case Study #14 ▬ Mary-Kate

Mary-Kate is a 25-year-old patient who was has been admitted into the hospital for drug overdose due to depression. On day 4 of her admission, her blood pressure dropped to 80/64, she developed breathlessness, and her urine output decreased to less than 30 mL/hr. The rapid response team was called due to the patient's deteriorating condition and the primary care provider (PCP) was notified. Mary-Kate had to be mechanically ventilated and placed in the medical intensive care unit.

Exercise 2-52: *Fill-in*

The nurse identifies these manifestations as _____.

Exercise 2-53: *Multiple-choice question*

A set of ABGs was completed before the patient was mechanically ventilated. The results were as follows: pH of 7.20, PaO_2 of 48, SaO_2 of 60%, $PaCO_2$ of 66, and a HCO_3 of 28. These results are indicative of:

    A. Metabolic acidosis

    B. Respiratory alkalosis

    C. Respiratory acidosis

    D. Metabolic alkalosis

 eResource 2-35: Use MedCalc's Acid–Base Online Calculator to verify your understanding: [Pathway: www.medcalc.com → select "Pulmonary" → select "ABG Calculator" and enter patient data]

Exercise 2-54: *Multiple-choice question*

What will be priority for the nurse after receiving this ABG result?

    A. Obtain a basic metabolic panel

    B. Administer oxygen

    C. Semi-Fowler position

    D. Obtain chest tube supplies

Answers to this chapter begin on page 67.

Exercise 2-55: *Select all that apply*

The nurse knows that potential risk factors for acute respiratory distress syndrome (ARDS) can include:

- ❏ Aspiration
- ❏ Sepsis
- ❏ Trauma
- ❏ Drug ingestion/overdose
- ❏ Smoke or toxic gas inhalation
- ❏ Exposure to an infected individual

e **eResource 2-36:** To learn more about treatment for ARDS, consult the Merck Manual: [Pathway: www.merckmanuals.com → select "The Merck Manual of Diagnosis and Therapy" → enter "ARDS" into the search field in the upper right corner → scroll down and select "Acute Hypoxemic Respiratory Failure" and scroll down to read "Etiology"]

Exercise 2-56: *Fill-in*

Mary-Kate is receiving lorazepam (Ativan) 0.5 mg to 1 mg IV as needed to minimize anxiety. What is the therapeutic effect of lorazepam?

_____

_____

e **eResource 2-37:** Consult Medscape on your mobile device to review the effect of this medication as well as safety and monitoring guidelines: [Pathway: Medscape → enter "lorazepam" into the search field and review content]

Unfolding Case Study #15 ▨ Anniston

Anniston is a 47-year-old patient who has been a smoker for 17 years. She has presented to the emergency department (ED) with complaints of hoarseness, difficulty swallowing, and chronic cough with rust-colored sputum.

Exercise 2-57: *Fill-in*

The nurse suspects that Anniston has_____.

The primary care provider has ordered a chest x-ray, basic metabolic panel (BMP), oxygen at 2 L/min per nasal cannula, Neupogen 5 mcg/kg subcutaneously daily, and Decadron 8 mg IV daily.

Exercise 2-58: *Calculation*

Calculate how many mcg of Neupogen will be given SC to Anniston who weighs 160 pounds.

_____

_____

Calculate how many mL of decadron Anniston will receive from a vial labeled dexamethasone 4 mg/mL.

_____

_____

eResource 2-38: To verify that these two drugs can be safely administered together, consult Epocrates on your mobile device: [Pathway: Epocrates → InteractionCheck → enter "Neupogen" and "Decadron" and view results]

Exercise 2-59: *Fill-in*
Identify at least three risk factors of lung cancer.

1. _____

2. _____

3. _____

The primary care provider has assessed Anniston and ordered three diagnostic procedures to identify the location of the lung cancer.

Exercise 2-60: *Fill-in*
Identify three diagnostic tests for lung cancer:

1. _____

2. _____

3. _____

Exercise 2-61: *Multiple-choice question*
The primary care provider has ordered a bronchoscopy. The client asks, "What is a bronchoscopy?" An appropriate response by the nurse is, "A bronchoscopy is:

    A. A needle that is inserted between three ribs and a piece of the tumor is burned."

    B. A set of x-rays that are taken that provide a four-dimensional picture of the lungs."

    C. A flexible tube that is inserted through your mouth and into your lungs to see the tumor and obtain a biopsy."

    D. Sound waves that are used to obtain pictures of the lungs to identify the tumors."

eResource 2-39: To learn more about this procedure, consult the Merck Manual: [Pathway: www.merckmanuals.com → select "The Merck Manual of Diagnosis and Therapy" → enter "brochoscopy" into the search field in the upper right corner → select "bronchoscopy" and review content]

The primary care provider has explained to Anniston that chemotherapy will be the treatment used for her lung cancer.

Answers to this chapter begin on page 67.

Exercise 2-62: *Fill-in*
Explain the purpose of chemotherapy for the treatment of cancer.

_____

_____

Exercise 2-63: *Fill-in*
Because Anniston will be receiving chemotherapy, the nurse should consider what five factors?

1. _____

2. _____

3. _____

4. _____

5. _____

Exercise 2-64: *Fill-in*
The nurse is to explain the importance of maintaining health while on chemotherapy. Identify three important factors in Anniston's chemotherapy education.

1. _____

2. _____

3. _____

eResource 2-40: To provide an overview of chemotherapy, the nurse shows Anniston several videos:
- *Chemotherapy Part 1*: http://youtu.be/eJq4xvjd_MU
- *Chemotherapy Part 2*: http://youtu.be/YzkAXSB3loM
- *Chemotherapy Part 3*: http://youtu.be/4BFSdj2iZTk
- *Chemotherapy Part 4*: http://youtu.be/QOts1ldjEYI

Answers to this chapter begin on page 67.

Answers

Exercise 2-1: *Fill-in*

The nurse suspects the diagnosis of **atelectasis**.

Exercise 2-2: *Fill-in*

Arterial blood gas results reveal a pH of 7.30, PCO_2 of 55, and HCO_3 of 26. What is this blood gas interpretation? **Respiratory acidosis**

Exercise 2-3: *Select all that apply*

The nurse identifies the following risk factors or manifestations of atelectasis:

☒ **Abdominal surgery—YES, this is a risk factor.**

☒ **Decreased or absent breath sounds—YES, this is a manifestation.**

❑ Equal chest movement—NO, there are unequal chest movements in patients with atelectasis.

☒ **Rapid heart rate—YES, this is a manifestation.**

☒ **Fever—YES, this is a manifestation.**

☒ **Confinement to bed—YES, this is a risk factor.**

Exercise 2-4: *Fill-in*

Victor's clinical manifestations require immediate intervention and assessment by the primary care provider. Identify at least three of Victor's clinical manifestations: **Diminished lung sounds, pulse of 126, and temperature 101.1°F.**

Exercise 2-5: *Fill-in*

The nurse informs Victor that his physical assessment findings require immediate testing to conclude atelectasis. What three ways can you diagnose atelectasis?

1. **Chest x-ray**
2. **Computed tomography (CT)**
3. **Manifestations of patient**

Exercise 2-6: *Select all that apply*

When educating patients about atelectasis, the nurse includes the following information:

☒ **Turn, cough, and deep breathe**

☒ **Incentive spirometry**

☒ **Chest percussion and postural drainage**

❑ Assess breath sounds every 12 hours

Exercise 2-7: *Multiple-choice question*

The nurse understands that Victor needs further teaching on the use of incentive spirometry when he states:

A. **"I only have to use it when I can't breathe."—YES, the use of incentive spirometry keeps your lungs active and clear, and will decrease the occurrence of shortness of breath**

B. "I am to use it every hour for 10 to 20 breaths while awake."—NO, this is true.

C. "I can continue to use it once I go home to keep my lungs clear."—NO, this is true.

D. "I am to hold the incentive spirometer in an upright position."—NO, this is true.

Exercise 2-8: *Fill-in*

Name three medications that can be used to treat atelectasis:

albuterol, Atrovent, Beconase-AQ.

Exercise 2-9: *Fill-in*

Based on the patient's symptoms, the nurse suspects William may have **pneumonia.**

Exercise 2-10: *Select all that apply*

The most common symptoms of pneumonia are:

☒ **Cough**

☒ **Fever**

☒ **Shaking chills**

☒ **Shortness of breath**

☒ **Weakness/fatigue**

☒ **Excessive sweating**

❑ Increased appetite

Exercise 2-11: *Select all that apply*

Based on William's symptoms, what increases his risk of pneumonia:

☒ **Older than 65**

☒ **Cigarette smoking**

☒ **Asthma**

☒ **Recent cold or flu**

❑ Pneumococcal vaccine every 5 years

Exercise 2-12: *Fill-in*

Identify at least three potential adverse effects of Levaquin:

1. **Rash**

2. **Nausea**

3. **Diarrhea**

Exercise 2-13: *Select all that apply*
After further education about Levaquin, the nurse asks William what medications he should be cautious of while taking Levaquin.

☒ **Antacids**

☒ **Magnesium**

☒ **Iron**

☒ **Zinc**

❏ Potassium

❏ Albuterol

Exercise 2-14: *Multiple-choice question*
After education of Levaquin, the nurse determines that William needs further instruction when he states:
A. "I will not drive until I know how this medication will affect me."—NO, this is true.
B. "I will stay out of the sun or use sunscreen."—NO, this is true and should be done.
C. **"I will take my Zantac at the same time as my Levaquin."—YES, these should not be taken at the same time.**
D. "If I have changes in my vision, I will notify my doctor."—No, this is true.

Exercise 2-15: *Fill-in*
Based on Caleb's physical assessment, he is exhibiting clinical manifestations of:
asthma

Exercise 2-16: *Fill-in*
The primary care provider has assessed Caleb and has ordered ABGs, chest x-ray, pulmonary function tests, and a sputum culture. Caleb's medical history includes smoker for 4 years, and a recent admission for asthma 3 weeks ago. Which test is the most accurate for diagnosing asthma and its severity? **Pulmonary function test**

Exercise 2-17: *Select all that apply*
Which of Caleb's manifestations can indicate a deterioration in his respiratory status?

☒ **SaO$_2$ of 88%**

☒ **Audible wheezing**

☒ **Tachypnea at 32 breaths/min**

☒ **Tachycardia at 118 beats/min**

❏ Age of 28

Exercise 2-18: *Fill-in*
Based on Caleb's manifestations, the nurse can expect to administer what classification of medication for his acute symptoms? **Bronchodilators**

Exercise 2-19: *Fill-in*

Identify three adverse effects of bronchodilators.

1. <u>**Restlessness**</u>
2. <u>**Nausea**</u>
3. <u>**Pallor**</u>

Exercise 2-20: *Fill-in*

After administering medication education to Caleb, name three nursing considerations that should be monitored?

1. <u>**Monitor for tachycardia**</u>
2. <u>**Monitor for tremors**</u>
3. <u>**Monitor for dry mouth**</u>

Exercise 2-21: *Select all that apply*

Potential irritants of asthma include:

☒ **House dust mites**

☒ **Mold or yeast spores**

☒ **Cat hair and saliva**

☒ **Cockroach particles**

☒ **Smoke**

☒ **Exercise**

Exercise 2-22: *Select all that apply*

Clinical manifestations of asthma include:

☒ **Increased respiratory rate**

☒ **Wheezing**

☒ **Productive cough**

☒ **Use of accessory muscles**

☒ **Dyspnea**

❏ Dry skin

Exercise 2-23: *Exhibit question*

Caleb's ABG result is as follows:

pH = 7.21

PO_2 = 66

PCO_2 = 55

HCO_3 = 22

Evaluate the ABG above and explain why it is occurring.

<u>**Respiratory acidosis is occurring because the lungs cannot remove the carbon dioxide the body has produced.**</u>

Exercise 2-24: *Matching*

Match the medication used to treat asthma in Column A to its effect in Column B.

Column A	Column B
A. Ventolin	__C__ Increases contraction of the diaphragm
B. Atrovent	__D__ Decreases airway inflammation
C. Theo-dur	__A__ Rapid relief of acute symptoms
D. Prednisone	__B__ Blocks the parasympathetic nervous system

Exercise 2-25: *Select all that apply*

Upon discharge from the emergency department, the nurse explains to Caleb that it is important that he maintains good health. Some positive patient outcomes for Caleb would include:

☒ **Decreases exposure to irritants**

☒ **Identifies mechanisms for coping**

☒ **Maintains adequate respiratory function**

❏ Not getting his family involved in his care

Exercise 2-26: *Fill-in*

Caleb is taught the importance of health promotion and disease prevention with asthma. What are three ways that can help Caleb improve his quality of life with asthma?

1. **Smoking cessation**
2. **Influenza and pneumonia vaccinations**
3. **Wear a protective mask when working in a environment with particles in the air**

Exercise 2-27: *Fill-in*

Identify four causes of COPD.

1. **Cigarette smoking**
2. **Allergies**
3. **Family history**
4. **Chronic respiratory tract infections**

Exercise 2-28: *Calculation*

Calculate aminophylline IV loading dose of 5 mg/kg over 30 minutes followed by 0.5 mg/kg/hr continuous intravenous. Calculate mL/hr to set the IV pump for the loading dose of aminophylline for Joshua who weighs 160 pounds. The aminophylline supply is 100 mg/100 mL D5W.

$$\frac{5 \text{ mg}}{\text{kg/30 min}} \quad \frac{100 \text{ mL}}{100 \text{ mg}} \quad \frac{1 \text{ kg}}{2.2 \text{ lb}} \quad \frac{160 \text{ lb}}{} \quad \frac{60 \text{ min}}{1 \text{ hr}} \quad \frac{5 \times 16 \times 6}{3 \times 2.2} = \frac{480}{6.6} = 72.7 \text{ mL/hr} = \textbf{73 mL/hr}$$

Exercise 2-29: *Calculation*

Calculate mL/hr to set the IV pump for the continuous dose of aminophylline for Joshua. The aminophylline is supplied as 1 g/250 mL D5W.

$$\frac{0.5 \text{ mg}}{\text{kg/hr}} \quad \frac{250 \text{ mL}}{1 \text{ g}} \quad \frac{1 \text{ g}}{1000 \text{ mg}} \quad \frac{1 \text{ kg}}{2.2 \text{ lb}} \quad \frac{160 \text{ lb}}{} \quad \frac{0.5 \times 25 \times 1 \times 16}{} = \frac{200}{22} = 9 \text{ mL/hr}$$

Exercise 2-30: *Fill-in*

What is the consideration of oxygen therapy in COPD patients?

Patients with COPD have a low partial pressure of oxygen in their blood. The use of supplementary oxygen can help improve the patient's condition; however, it can also elevate carbon dioxide in the blood, which can be toxic to the body.

Exercise 2-31: *Multiple-choice question*

Joshua's ABG results revealed a pH of 7.30, PaO_2 of 50, PCO_2 of 48, and a HCO_3 of 26. What is Joshua's ABG interpretation?

A. Metabolic alkalosis—NO, the pH is low.

B. Respiratory acidosis—YES

C. Metabolic acidosis—NO, HCO_3 is normal.

D. Respiratory alkalosis—NO, the pH is low.

Exercise 2-32: *Fill-in*

What classification of medications will be administered to Joshua to relieve his symptoms?

1. **Beta-agonist bronchodilators (albuterol)**
2. **Anticholingeric bronchodilators (Atrovent)**
3. **Corticosteroids (Beconase-AQ)**

Exercise 2-33: *Fill-in*

Identify two types of breathing techniques to control Joshua's dyspneic episodes.

1. **Pursed-lip breathing**
2. **Diaphragmatic breathing or abdominal breathing**

Exercise 2-34: *Fill-in*

Incentive spirometry is used to monitor Joshua's lung expansion. What education is given to the patient in regard to how to use the incentive spirometry?

Instruct the patient to keep a tight mouth seal around the spirometer mouthpiece and inhale and hold the breath for 3 to 5 seconds. This promotes lung expansion in the patient.

Exercise 2-35: *Select all that apply*

The nurse knows that promoting adequate nutrition is important while Joshua is in the hospital. What education is given to Joshua on the importance of nutrition?

☒ **Encourage 2 to 3 L/day of fluid**

☒ **Aids in the prevention of infection**

☒ **High-calorie and high-protein diet**

☐ Consume caffeine

☒ **Avoid caffeine**

Exercise 2-36: *Fill-in*

While in the hospital, other interdisciplinary care teams have been consulted for Joshua. What is the importance of respiratory services, nutritional services, and rehabilitative care?

Respiratory services: **Administer breathing treatments and airway management**

Nutritional services: **Contacted for weight loss or gain related to diagnosis or medication**

Rehabilitative services: **Consulted for prolonged weakness or when patient needs assistance in activities of daily living**

Exercise 2-37: *Select all that apply*

Upon discharge from the hospital, what education is given to Joshua to improve his quality of care since his diagnosis of COPD?

☒ **Encourage smoking cessation**

☒ **Encourage influenza and pneumonia vaccines**

☒ **Promote hand hygiene to prevent infection**

☐ Discontinue medications once feeling better

☒ **Report fluid retention and weight gain**

Exercise 2-38: *Fill-in*

The nurse suspects Patterson of having a **pulmonary embolism.**

Exercise 2-39: *Select all that apply*

Risk factors associated with pulmonary embolism include:

☒ **Pregnancy**

☒ **Tobacco use**

☒ **Oral contraceptive and estrogen therapy**

☐ Decreased platelet count

☒ **Long-term immobility**

Exercise 2-40: *Fill-in*

What is the significance in ordering a chest x-ray and a V/Q scan?

A chest x-ray provides initial identification of a pulmonary embolism and a V/Q scan shows the circulation of air and blood in the lungs and can detect a pulmonary embolism.

Exercise 2-41: *Fill-in*

What does the positive D-dimer signify to the nurse and the primary care provider?

It signifies there may be a blood clot (thrombus) formation.

Exercise 2-42: *Fill-in*

What three types of anticoagulant medications can be administered for pulmonary embolism?

1. **Enoxaparin (Lovenox)**
2. **Heparin**
3. **Warfarin (Coumadin)**

Exercise 2-43: *Calculation*

Calculate how many mL of heparin Patterson will receive IV from a multidose vial labeled 10,000 units/mL.

$$\frac{5000 \text{ units}}{} \quad \frac{\text{mL}}{10,000 \text{ units}} \quad \frac{5}{10} = 0.5 \text{ mL}$$

Calculate mL/hr to set the IV pump for the continuous dose of heparin. Heparin is supplied as 25,000 units/250 mL D5W.

$$\frac{1000 \text{ units}}{\text{hr}} \quad \frac{250 \text{ mL}}{25,000 \text{ units}} \quad 10 = 10 \text{ mL/hr}$$

Exercise 2-44: *Select all that apply*

What type of education is given to Patterson in the treatment and prevention of a pulmonary embolism?

☒ **Promote smoking cessation**

☒ **Encourage wearing of compression stockings to promote circulation**

☒ **Avoid crossing legs**

☒ **Avoid long periods of immobility**

❏ Discourage physical activity such as walking

Exercise 2-45: *Fill-in*

Upon discharge from the hospital, the nurse should instruct Patterson on increased risk for bruising and bleeding while on anticoagulants. What should Patterson know? **Avoid taking aspirin products unless directed by a doctor. Monitor skin and mouth daily for bleeding and bruising. Use electric shavers and soft-bristled toothbrushes. Don't blow your nose hard; if it should bleed, apply light pressure.**

Exercise 2-46: *Multiple-choice question*

After discharge education has been completed, the nurse knows that Patterson needs further instructions when she states:
A. "I will adhere to anticoagulant therapy."—NO, this is correct.
B. "I will wear my compression stockings to promote circulation."—NO, this should be done.
C. "I will only smoke three times a week."—YES, she needs to quit smoking.
D. "I will check my mouth and skin daily for bleeding and bruising."—NO, this should be done.

Exercise 2-47: *Fill-in*

What does the nurse suspect Martha's subjective and objective data results mean she has?
Pulmonary edema

Exercise 2-48: *Fill-in*

Identify three of Martha's risk factors for pulmonary edema.
  1. **Myocardial infarction**
  2. **Hypertension**
  3. **Left-sided heart failure**

Exercise 2-49: *Fill-in*

The primary care provider has ordered two diuretics, furosemide (Lasix) and bumetanide (Bumex), to alleviate fluid overload. What does the nurse know about these medications?
They are rapid-acting diuretics that promote fluid excretion in the body.

Exercise 2-50: *Select all that apply*

What type of nursing care is imperative for Martha in order to achieve positive health outcomes?
☒ **Monitor intake and output**
❑ Maintain intravenous fluids
☒ **Maintain a patent airway**
☒ **Restrict fluid intake**
☒ **Monitor hourly urine output**

Exercise 2-51: *Fill-in*

Upon discharge, the nurse will educate Martha on the importance of health promotion and disease prevention for pulmonary edema. What type of information can be taught? **Consume a low-sodium diet and restrict fluids by mouth. Encourage smoking cessation. Continue medication regimen unless directed differently by the doctor. Encourage activity.**

Exercise 2-52: *Fill-in*

The nurse identifies these manifestations as **acute respiratory distress syndrome.**

Exercise 2-53: *Multiple-choice question*

A set of ABGs were done before the patient was mechanically ventilated. The results were as follows: pH of 7.20, PaO_2 of 48, SaO_2 of 60%, $PaCO_2$ of 66, and a HCO_3 of 28. These results are indicative of:

A. Metabolic acidosis—NO, the HCO_3 is high.

B. Respiratory alkalosis—NO, the pH is low.

C. Respiratory acidosis—YES

D. Metabolic alkalosis—NO, the pH is low.

Exercise 2-54: *Multiple-choice question*

What will be priority for the nurse after receiving this ABG result?

A. Obtain a basic metabolic panel—NO, although this is good to have it is not the priority.

B. Administer oxygen—YES, the patient is lacking O_2.

C. Semi-Fowler position—NO, this position does not provide adequate support for a ventilated patient.

D. Obtain chest tube supplies—NO, this is not indicated at this time.

Exercise 2-55: *Select all that apply*

The nurse knows that potential risk factors for acute respiratory distress syndrome (ARDS) can include:

☒ **Aspiration**

☒ **Sepsis**

☒ **Trauma**

☒ **Drug ingestion/overdose**

☒ **Smoke or toxic gas inhalation**

❏ Exposure to an infected individual

Exercise 2-56: *Select all that apply*

Mary-Kate is receiving lorazepam (Ativan) 0.5 mg to 1 mg IV to minimize anxiety. What is the therapeutic effect of lorazepam (Ativan)?

The therapeutic effect of lorazepam causes mild suppression of REM sleep, while increasing total sleep time.

Exercise 2-57: *Fill-in*

The nurse suspects that Anniston has **lung cancer.**

Exercise 2-58: *Calculation*

Calculate how many mcg of Neupogen will be given subcuanteously to Anniston who weighs 160 pounds.

$$\frac{5 \text{ mcg}}{\text{kg}} \quad \frac{1 \text{ kg}}{2.2 \text{ lb}} \quad \frac{160 \text{ lb}}{} \quad \frac{5 \times 1}{2.2} \quad \frac{160 \times 800}{2.2} = 363.6 \text{ mcg or 364 mcg}$$

Calculate how many mL of Decadron Anniston will receive from a vial labeled dexamethasone 4 mg/mL.

$$\frac{8 \text{ mg}}{} \quad \frac{\text{mL}}{4 \text{ mg}} \quad \frac{8}{4} = 2 \text{ mL}$$

Exercise 2-59: *Fill-in*

Identify at least three risk factors for lung cancer.

1. **Cigarette smoker**
2. **Exposure to radiation**
3. **Exposed to inhaled environmental irritants**

Exercise 2-60: *Fill-in*

Identify three diagnostic tests for lung cancer:

1. **Chest x-ray**
2. **Computed tomography (CT)**
3. **Bronchoscopy**

Exercise 2-61: *Multiple-choice question*

The primary care provider has ordered a bronchoscopy. The client asks, "What is a bronchoscopy?" An appropriate response by the nurse is, "A bronchoscopy is:

A. A needle that is inserted between three ribs and a piece of the tumor is burned."— NO, this is not accurate.

B. A set of x-rays that are taken that provide a four-dimensional picture of the lungs."—NO, this is not accurate.

C. **A flexible tube that is inserted through your mouth and into your lungs to see the tumor and obtain a biopsy."—YES, this is what the scope does.**

D. Sound waves that are used to obtain sectional pictures of the lungs to identify the tumors."—NO, this is not accurate.

Exercise 2-62: *Fill-in*

Explain the purpose of chemotherapy for the treatment of lung cancer.

Chemotherapy destroys cancer cells as well as healthy cells to prevent DNA formation.

Exercise 2-63: *Fill-in*

Because Anniston will be receiving chemotherapy, the nurse should consider what five factors?

1. **Monitor for nausea and vomiting**
2. **Monitor for fatigue**
3. **Assess for shortness of breath**
4. **Assess for mouth and throat lesions**
5. **Assess for decreased immune function**

Exercise 2-64: *Fill-in*

The nurse is to explain the importance of maintaining health while on chemotherapy. Identify three important factors in Anniston's chemotherapy education.

1. **Encourage oral hygiene**
2. **Inform the patient of persistent nausea and vomiting**
3. **Inform the patient about hair loss (alopecia), which usually occurs 7 to 10 days after chemotherapy treatment**

3

Nursing Care of the Patient With Renal Disease

Rhonda M. Brogdon

Unfolding Case Study #16 ▢ Julia

Julia is a 55-year-old patient who has come to her primary care provider (PCP) complaining of leakage of urine. She stated, "It happens when I laugh or sneeze." Julia further states that it is "embarrassing when she is around people." Julia has a history of six vaginal births, a past stroke, and hypertension, and is 5 feet 5 inches and weighs 220 pounds. Julia also takes Norvasc 10 mg by mouth twice a day and Lasix 40 mg twice a day.

Exercise 3-1: *Fill-in*

Based on Julia's signs and symptoms, the primary care provider suspects:

_____.

Julia is upset that this is happening to her because she feels that she just got her life back after her stroke. The PCP explains to Julia that there are contributing risk factors that occur that may cause incontinence.

Exercise 3-2: *Fill-in*

What contributing risk factors does Julia have?

1. _____

2. _____

3. _____

4. _____

5. _____

6. _____

eResource 3-1: To supplement your understanding of the risk factors, refer to Epocrates Online: [Pathway: http://online.epocrates.com → enter "incontinence" into the search field → select "urinary incontinence" → select "risk factors" and review content]

The PCP explains to Julia that there are six major types of urinary incontinence.

Exercise 3-3: *Fill-in*
What are the six major types of urinary incontinence?

1. _____

2. _____

3. _____

4. _____

5. _____

6. _____

Julia does not understand the types of urinary incontinence. The PCP explains each type to Julia.

Exercise 3-4: *Matching*
Match the type of urinary incontinence in Column A to its definition in Column B.

Column A	Column B
A. Stress	_____ Inability to get to the toilet to urinate
B. Urge	_____ Involuntary loss of urine that does not respond generally to treatment
C. Overflow	_____ Loss of small amounts of urine when coughing, sneezing or laughing
D. Functional	_____ Involuntary loss of a moderate amount of urine usually without warning
E. Reflex	_____ Inability to stop urine flow long enough to reach toilet
F. Total incontinence	_____ Urinary retention associated with bladder overdistension

 eResource 3-2: For more information regarding the types and etiology of urinary incontinence, refer to Medscape on your mobile device: [Pathway: Medscape → enter "incontinence" into the search field → select "urinary incontinence" and review content under the "overview" tab]

Answers to this chapter begin on page 95.

Julia's PCP has ordered diagnostic testing for urinary incontinence. The PCP has ordered a postvoid residual urine, urinalysis and urine culture/sensitivity, serum creatinine and blood urea nitrogen (BUN), and an ultrasound of the bladder.

Exercise 3-5: *Fill-in*
Explain the significance of each of these tests as it relates to urinary incontinence.

1. Postvoid residual urine: _____
2. Urinalysis and urine culture/sensitivity: _____
3. Serum creatinine and BUN: _____
4. Ultrasound of the bladder: _____

 cResource 3-3: To learn more about the diagnostic testing ordered for Julia, refer to Medscape on your mobile device: [Pathway: Medscape → enter "urinary incontinence" into the search field → select "workup" and review all the diagnostic procedures]

Exercise 3-6: *Select all that apply*
Which of the following interventions can control or eliminate Julia's incontinence?

❑ Minimize delays in toileting

❑ Perform Kegel exercises

❑ Take prescribed diuretics in morning/mid-afternoon

❑ Increase fluid intake at bedtime

❑ Bladder retraining

 eResource 3-4: To learn more about the recommended treatment and management for urinary incontinence, refer to:
■ Medscape on your mobile device: [Pathway: Medscape → enter "urinary incontinence" into the search field → select "treatment and management" and review content]
■ Merck Manual: [Pathway: www.merckmanuals.com → select "Merck Manual for Health Care Professionals" → enter "urinary incontinence" into the search field → select "treatment" and review content]

Exercise 3-7: *Multiple-choice question*
The nurse knows the best nursing diagnosis for Julia will be:

A. Pain

B. Activity intolerance

C. Impaired urinary elimination

D. Self-care deficit

eResource 3-5: To learn more about management of urinary incontinence in women to guide development of a nursing care plan for Julia, refer to *Urinary Incontinence Treatments for Women (Beyond the Basics):* http://goo.gl/nleHm

Answers to this chapter begin on page 95.

Unfolding Case Study #17 ▨ Simone

Simone is a 29-year-old patient who presents to the emergency department (ED) with a complaint of frequent urination and burning along with pain when she does urinate. She thinks she may have seen blood in her urine but was not sure. Simone has also complained of perineal itching and an unpleasant odor of her urine. Simone takes prescribed oral contraceptives, has never been pregnant, and is sexually active.

Exercise 3-8: *Fill-in*
The nurse suspects Simone of having a _____.

Exercise 3-9: *Fill-in*
What presenting signs and symptoms indicate urinary tract infection for Simone?

1. _____

2. _____

3. _____

4. _____

5. _____

e **eResource 3-6:** To learn more about the clinical presentation of a urinary tract infection, consult Epocrates Online: [Pathway: http://online .epocrates.com → select the "diseases" tab → enter "urinary tract infection" into the search field → review "Key Highlights" and "History and Exam" details]

Exercise 3-10: *Fill-in*
The primary care provider has ordered an urinalysis and urine culture and sensitivity for Simone. Expected findings of the diagnostic testing will include:

_____

The primary care provider (PCP) has prescribed Macrobid 100 mg every 12 hours after meals for 7 days and Bactrim DS one tablet twice a day for 3 days after reviewing the results of the urinalysis and urine culture and sensitivity.

Exercise 3-11: *Fill-in*
Name four side effects of Bactrim DS.

1. _____

2. _____

3. _____

4. _____

Answers to this chapter begin on page 95.

eResource 3-7: To reinforce your understanding of the effects of Bactrim DS, consult:
- Epocrates on your mobile device: [Pathway: Epocrates → enter "Bactrim" into the search field → select "Bactrim DS" → scroll down to review "Adverse Reactions" and review "serious reactions" and "common reactions"]
- Skyscape's RxDrugs: [Pathway: RxDrugs → enter "Bactrim" into the search field → select " Bactrim DS" → scroll down to review "Adverse Reactions"]

Exercise 3-12: *Select all that apply*

The nurse is explaining to Simone what she should expect with Macrobid. What should Simone expect to happen or expect to see with Macrobid?

❏ Reddish/brown discoloration of urine

❏ Abdominal pain

❏ Photosensitivity

❏ Nausea/vomiting

❏ Bulimia

 eResource 3-8: To reinforce your understanding of the effects of Macrobid consult:
- Epocrates on your mobile device: [Pathway: Epocrates → enter "Macrobid" into the search field → select "Macrobid" → scroll down to review "Adverse Reactions" and review "serious reactions" and "common reactions"]
- Skyscape's RxDrugs: [Pathway: RxDrugs → enter "Macrobid" into the search field → select "Macrobid" → scroll down to review "Adverse Reactions"]

Exercise 3-13: *Select all that apply*

The nurse is providing discharge teaching to Simone. What types of interventions will help Simone to decrease the risk of another urinary tract infection?

❏ Urinate before and after intercourse

❏ Avoid wearing tight clothing

❏ Wipe the perineal area from front to back

❏ Discourage fluid intake

❏ Take all prescribed medications

❏ Avoid use of products containing perfumes

 eResource 3-9: To learn more about prevention of urinary tract infections among women, consult Medscape on your mobile device: [Pathway: Medscape → enter "urinary" into the search field → select "Prevention of Urinary Tract Infections in Women" and review content]

Answers to this chapter begin on page 95.

Unfolding Case Study #18 ▨ Grayson

Grayson, a 40-year-old patient, presented to the emergency department (ED) complaining of pain in his left lower quadrant. He describes his pain on a numerical scale of 0 to 10 as 10, the highest pain rating. Grayson states that his pain is sharp and constant and has radiated to his left flank. Grayson denies dysuria and hematuria; however, he does complain of nausea with no vomiting. His vital signs are temperature 98.8°F, pulse of 90, respirations 22, and blood pressure of 146/88. He has a medical history of allergies, pneumonia, and hypertension and no surgical history.

Exercise 3-14: *Fill-in*

The primary care provider suspects a diagnosis of _____.

Grayson does not understand how he got kidney stones. The primary care provider (PCP) tells Grayson that urolithiasis is the presence of calculi (stones) in the urinary tract. Urolithiasis can be caused by several factors.

Exercise 3-15: *Select all that apply*

What can contribute to the formation of renal calculi?

❑ Infection

❑ Prolonged acidic or alkaline urine

❑ Increased intake of calcium or oxalate-rich foods

❑ Decreased urine production

❑ Decreased intake of calcium or oxalate-rich foods

ⓔ **eResource 3-10:** To learn more about factors contributing to the formation of renal calculi, refer to:
▪ Epocrates Online: [Pathway: http://online.epocrates.com → enter "renal calculi" into the search field → select "risk factors" and review content]
▪ Merck Manual: [Pathway: www.merckmanuals.com → select "Merck Manual for Health Care Professionals" → enter "renal calculi" into the search field → select "urinary calculi" → review "etiology" and "pathophysiology." Be sure to look at all the images]

Grayson is still complaining of severe pain in his left lower quadrant. The primary care provider has ordered morphine 10 mg intravenously (IV) STAT and 4 mg IV every 4 hours as needed for pain, continuous IV fluids of normal saline at 150 mL/hr, computed tomographic (CT) scan of abdomen without contrast, urinalysis/urine culture, calcium and phosphorus blood levels, and a complete blood count (CBC).

ⓔ **eResource 3-11:** To reinforce your understanding of morphine, its indication and effects, consult on your mobile device:
▪ Medscape: [Pathway: Medscape → enter "Morphine" into the search field → review content]
▪ Skyscape's RxDrugs [Pathway: RxDrugs → enter "Morphine" into the search field → review content]

Answers to this chapter begin on page 95.

■ Epocrates: [Pathway: Epocrates → enter "Morphine" into the search field → review content]

Exercise 3-16: *Fill-in*

The primary care provider knows that the key symptom of urolithiasis is _____.

 eResource 3-12: To reinforce your understanding of the key findings accompanying urolithiasis, consult Epocrates Online: [Pathway: http://online.epocrates.com → enter "urolithiasis" into the search field → review "key findings"]

The urinalysis results revealed a high specific gravity level, microscopic hematuria, crystals, casts, and pyuria.

Exercise 3-17: *Multiple-choice question*

Grayson asks the primary care provider, "What is a cast?" The primary care provider replies:

    A. Fatty deposits in the urine

    B. Glucose in the urine

    C. A type of tumor

    D. Cylinder particles made of white/red blood cells formed in the renal tubules

Exercise 3-18: *Multiple-choice question*

What is the pathophysiologic reason for Grayson's nausea?

    A. Gallbladder hematoma

    B. Dysphagia

    C. Severe pain

    D. Metabolic alkalosis

 eResource 3-13: To learn more about the symptoms associated with urolithiasis (urinary calculi), consult Merck Manual: [Pathway: www.merckmanuals.com → select "Merck Manual for Health Care Professionals" → enter "urolithiasis" (or "renal caluli") into the search field → scroll down to "symptoms and signs" and "diagnosis" to review content]

Exercise 3-19: *Multiple-choice question*

Which of the following can contribute to the formation of renal calculi?

    A. Hypothyroidism

    B. Changes in urine pH

    C. Hypotension

    D. Hypocalcemia

 eResource 3-14: To learn more about renal calculi formation, review the brief video, *Renal Calculi*: http://goo.gl/roXgW

The CT scan of the abdomen revealed two small renal calculi that were approximately 5 mm in diameter. The PCP wanted to promote passage of the calculi before taking an invasive method. The nurse brought in a urine strainer and educated him on its purpose and also encouraged Grayson to drink fluids.

Answers to this chapter begin on page 95.

Exercise 3-20: *Multiple-choice question*

Which statement by Grayson lets the nurse know that he understands the purpose of a urine strainer?

    A. "The urine strainer is to be used only when I have pain."

    B. "The urine strainer is to strain all my urine for collection of the calculi."

    C. "The urine strainer is for my guests to use that visit me."

    D. "The urine strainer is used to measure my urine output."

The nurse knows that Grayson is at risk for developing a urinary tract infection (UTI).

Exercise 3-21: *Fill-in*

Why does the presence of renal calculi put Grayson at risk for a UTI?

_____

_____

The nurse provided dietary education to Grayson to help decrease the formation of renal calculi.

Exercise 3-22: *Multiple-choice question*

Which foods should Grayson have a low intake of?

    A. White potatoes/bananas

    B. Peanut butter/milk

    C. Legumes/fish

    D. Fish/chicken

 eResource 3-15: To supplement patient teaching, the nurse shows Grayson MedlinePlus's interactive tutorial about kidney stones: [Pathway: www.nlm.nih.gov/medlineplus → enter "kidney stones" into the search field → select "kidney stones interactive tutorial" and view content (or use quick link: http://goo.gl/HdBah)]

Grayson has successfully passed his stones without surgical intervention. His pain has been decreased to a 4 on a numerical pain scale of 0 to 10, with 10 being the highest.

Exercise 3-23: *Select all that apply*

What education is provided to Grayson before his discharge?

    ❏ Follow prescribed dietary and medication regimens

    ❏ Encourage increased fluid intake

    ❏ Report signs and symptoms of pain

    ❏ Report the inability to void

    ❏ Hematuria is a normal finding

Answers to this chapter begin on page 95.

eResource 3-16: To supplement Grayson's discharge teaching, the nurse provides information regarding dietary measures to prevent kidney stone formation by providing the National Kidney and Urologic Diseases Information Clearinghouse (NKUDIC), *Diet for Kidney Stone Prevention*: http://goo.gl/9lbli

Unfolding Case Study #19 ▨ Kimberly

Kimberly is a 35-year-old patient who was admitted to the hospital with a complaint of nausea for 1 week with minimal abdominal pain. She rated her pain a 3 on a numeric scale of 0 to 10, with 10 being the highest. Today, she has experienced vomiting, and stated, "I just feel really bad." Kimberly also stated, "I have not had an appetite." Her medical history is significant for hypertension for 5 years, anemia, and a hysterectomy. Kimberly's vital signs are temperature 98.9°F, pulse of 108, respirations of 22, and a blood pressure of 150/90, and 2+ pitting edema in ankles. Her home medications include Norvasc 10 mg once a day, metoprolol 100 mg once a day, and ferrous sulfate 325 mg once a day. The primary care provider (PCP) has examined Kimberly and has ordered a metabolic panel. The results are shown in Table 3-1:

Table 3-1: Laboratory Results

Blood Lab Value	Patient Value	Normal Range
Sodium	150	135–145 mEq/L
Potassium	5.9	3.5–5.0 mEq/L
Chloride	119	97–107 mEq/L
Glucose	130	60–110 mg/dL
Calcium	7.3	8.5–10.5 mg/dL
CO_2	14.0	20–30 mEq/L
Phosphorus	10.4	2.3–4.3 mg/dL
Blood pH	7.32	7.38–7.42
BUN (blood urea nitrogen)	59	7–24 mg/dL
Creatinine	10.0	0.6–1.2 mg/dL

 eResource 3-17: To review normal serum blood levels, refer to:
▨ Epocrates Online: [Pathway: http://online.epocrates.com → select "Tables" tab → scroll down and select "Lab Reference" and review content]
▨ Global RPh: http://goo.gl/BrHnj

Exercise 3-24: *Fill-in*
Based on Kimberly's signs/symptoms and metabolic results, the primary care provider is concerned about what pathophysiological process? _____.

Answers to this chapter begin on page 95.

Exercise 3-25: *Multiple-choice question*
According to the metabolic results, what two lab values reflect the ability of the kidney to excrete waste?

        A. Sodium and chloride

        B. Potassium and BUN

        C. BUN and creatinine

        D. Creatinine and sodium

 eResource 3-18: To reinforce your understanding of the normal function of the kidneys, view *Urinary System Part 1—The Kidneys:* http://youtu.be/zEpUQkQ-uKM

Upon further evaluation of the metabolic results, the PCP notes that the electrolyte values show a diminished capacity of Kimberly's kidneys to regulate acid–base balance.

Exercise 3-26: *Multiple-choice question*
What acid–base balance process is occurring?

        A. Respiratory acidosis

        B. Metabolic acidosis

        C. Respiratory alkalosis

        D. Metabolic alkalosis

Exercise 3-27: *Fill-in*
Why is this acid–base process occurring?

_____

_____

Exercise 3-28: *Fill-in*
The primary care provider is also concerned that Kimberly's potassium level is 5.9 mEq/L. What is the pathophysiological process that is causing the elevation?

_____

_____

Exercise 3-29: *Multiple-choice question*
An elevated potassium level poses what immediate danger to Kimberly?

        A. Disrupts the heart's conduction system

        B. Disrupts the lungs' exchange of air

        C. Disrupts the gastrointestinal system

        D. Disrupts the integumentary system

Answers to this chapter begin on page 95.

The primary care provider has ordered a urinalysis. The results are shown in Table 3-2:

Table 3-2: Urinalysis Results

Urinalysis Value	Patient Values	Normal Values
Protein	3 gm/dL	Absent
Specific gravity	1.007	1.005–1.030
pH	5.2	5.5–6.5 (average range)
Glucose	Present (2+)	Absent
Blood (hemoglobin)	3+	Absent
Casts	Granular and epithelial cells 3–8 p/lpf	Absent or rare
White blood cells	5–15 p/hpf	0–1 p/hpf
Red blood cells	6–15 p/hpf	Rare
Epithelial cells (renal)	30–50 p/hpf	0–3 p/hpf

p/lpf = per low-power field; p/hpf = per high-power field.

Exercise 3-30: *Fill-in*

The urinalysis shows the presence of glucose and protein in the urine. What does this mean?

Exercise 3-31: *Multiple-choice question*

The results of the urinalysis indicate the presence of casts. What damage do casts cause to the kidneys?

    A. Damage to the urethra

    B. Damage to the tubules

    C. Damage to the bladder

    D. Damage to the anal orifice

Exercise 3-32: *Select all that apply*

What urinalysis results indicate acute renal failure?

❑ Protein

❑ Cells

❑ Casts

❑ Specific gravity

❑ pH

❑ Glucose

Answers to this chapter begin on page 95.

eResource 3-19: To learn more about the clinical presentation of acute renal failure and diagnostic procedure, consult:
- Epocrates Online: [Pathway: http://online.epocrates.com → enter "acute renal failure" into the search field → review "Key Highlights" and "History & Exam"]
- Merck Manual: [Pathway: www.merckmanuals.com → select "Merck Manual for Health Care Professionals" → enter "acute renal failure" into the search field → select "acute renal failure" and review "overview" and "symptoms & signs"]

eResource 3-20: To better understand acute renal failure, watch the following brief lectures by Dr. Roger Seheult entitled *Acute Renal Failure Explained Clearly!*:
- Part 1: http://goo.gl/MPV91
- Part 2: http://goo.gl/LXyfA
- Part 3: http://goo.gl/udfTY

A nephrologist was consulted based on the metabolic and urinalysis results. The nephrologist wanted to challenge Kimberly's kidneys by diuresis. Kimberly was started on normal saline at 150 mL/hr and IV Lasix 100 mg every 12 hours and Kayexalate 30 g was given STAT for the elevated potassium level.

Exercise 3-33: *Fill-in*
What is the purpose of diuresis in treating acute kidney failure?

_____

_____

Kimberly's urinalysis result is positive for protein. The nephrologist has explained the importance of maintaining a low-protein, potassium/phosphorus diet and also consulted the dietician for further education.

Exercise 3-34: *Fill-in*
Why is protein restricted in Kimberly's diet?

_____

_____

eResource 3-21: For material to supplement the diet teaching for Kimberly, consult:
- Virgina Commonwealth University Health System's *The Renal Diet*: http://goo.gl/7WixQ
- MedlinePlus's *Diet: Chronic Kidney Disease:* http://goo.gl/BJz3J

Kimberly's acute renal failure was stabilized through diuresis and she did not have to require renal dialysis.

Answers to this chapter begin on page 95.

Exercise 3-35: *Fill-in*
What is renal dialysis?

_____

_____

If Kimberly had required renal dialysis, she had the options of hemodialysis and peritoneal dialysis.

Exercise 3-36: *Fill-in*
What is hemodialysis?

_____

_____

What is peritoneal dialysis?

_____

_____

eResource 3-22: To learn more about peritoneal dialysis and hemodialysis, view the following videos:
- Peritoneal Dialysis: http://goo.gl/oOpnq
- Hemodialysis: http://goo.gl/x3VHI

eResource 3-23: To learn more about dialysis fistulas and peritoneal dialysis, refer to Medscape on your mobile device: [Pathway: Medscape → enter "dialysis" into the search field → select "dialysis fistulas" and review content then select "peritoneal dialysis catheter insertion" and review content]

Unfolding Case Study #20 ▨ Ethan

Ethan is a 50-year-old patient who has presented to the emergency department (ED) with a blood glucose result of 160 and a blood pressure of 180/100. He has no complaints of pain or shortness of breath. His lower extremities have +1 pitting edema, and a right-arm dialysis graft with a positive bruit and thrill. He has a history of hypertension and diabetes mellitus for 10 years and chronic renal failure, and he receives hemodialysis treatment 3 days a week on Monday, Wednesday, and Friday. He receives lisinopril 40 mg twice a day, Norvasc 10 mg once a day, and metoprolol 50 mg once a day. Ethan's blood glucose has been maintained by diet and exercise.

Exercise 3-37: *Fill-in*
What is chronic renal failure?

_____

_____

Answers to this chapter begin on page 95.

Exercise 3-38: *Fill-in*

Explain the five stages of chronic renal failure.

Stage I: _____

Stage II: _____

Stage III: _____

Stage IV: _____

Stage V: _____

Exercise 3-39: *Select all that apply*

What are some symptoms of chronic renal disease?

❑ Shortness of breath

❑ Fatigue or weakness

❑ Increase in appetite

❑ Nausea/vomiting

❑ Urine output greater than 400 mL/day

e **eResource 3-24:** To learn more about the presentation of chronic renal disease, refer to Epocrates Online: [Pathway: http://online.epocrates.com → select "diseases" tab → enter "renal disease" → review content under "Clinical Presentation"]

Exercise 3-40: *Select all that apply*

What risk factors for chronic renal failure does Ethan present with?

❑ Diabetes mellitus

❑ Hypertension

❑ Drug toxicity

❑ Renal tuberculosis

❑ Congenital disorder

Exercise 3-41: *Multiple-choice question*

Ethan's blood glucose is within an acceptable range. His urinalysis was positive for blood and protein. What complication of diabetes might be occurring?

A. Hepatorenal syndrome

B. Chronic renal failure related to diabetic nephropathy

C. Acute renal failure related to urolithiasis

D. Scleroderma

e **eResource 3-25:** To learn about the long-term management of chronic renal failure, consult Medscape on your mobile device: [Pathway: Medscape → enter "dialysis" into the search field → select "Dialysis Complications of Chronic Renal Failure" and review content]

Answers to this chapter begin on page 95.

Exercise 3-42: *Multiple-choice question*

What is generally the first sign of renal dysfunction in a diabetic patient?

- A. Proteinuria
- B. Hyperkalemia
- C. Hyperparathyroidism
- D. Wilms's tumor

Ethan stated that he missed his dialysis treatment on Friday. The primary care provider (PCP) has called the on-call dialysis nurse to administer dialysis.

Exercise 3-43: *Select all that apply*

What are some acute complications that may occur during Ethan's treatment?

- ❏ Muscle cramps
- ❏ Angina
- ❏ Hypotension
- ❏ Arrhythmias
- ❏ Cardiac arrest
- ❏ Bowel perforation

The dialysis nurse must assess the graft for a thrill and bruit before beginning the treatment.

Exercise 3-44: *Fill-in*

Why must the nurse assess the graft for a thrill and bruit?

_____

_____

The nurse knows that graft access sites present complications for the dialysis patient.

Exercise 3-45: *Fill-in*

What are the two most common complications of a dialysis graft access?

1. _____
2. _____

After Ethan's dialysis treatment, his blood pressure decreased to 140/88 and the pitting edema in his lower extremities was alleviated.

Exercise 3-46: *Select all that apply*

What is included in the aftercare by the nurse?

- ❏ Monitor vascular access site for bleeding
- ❏ Auscultate the thrill and palpate the bruit
- ❏ Auscultate the bruit and palpate the thrill
- ❏ Vascular access site only used for treatment
- ❏ How to apply a dressing to graft site if bleeding occurs

Answers to this chapter begin on page 95.

Exercise 3-47: *Multiple-choice question*

Ethan is being prepared for discharge to home. The nurse knows that Ethan needs further discharge instructions with this statement:

    A. "I will keep my graft site clean and dry."

    B. "I will notify the primary care provider if I have swelling, redness, or drainage at my graft site."

    C. "I can take my blood pressure in the same arm as my graft site."

    D. "I must avoid excessive pressure on my graft arm site."

 eResource 3-26: To supplement the patient teaching, refer to *Hemodialysis Shunt, Graft, and Fistula Care*: http://goo.gl/50G5t

Answers

Exercise 3-1: *Fill-in*

Based on Julia's signs and symptoms, the primary care provider suspects:

urinary incontinence

Exercise 3-2: *Fill-in*

What contributing risk factors does Julia have?

1. **Vaginal births**
2. **Obesity**
3. **Stroke**
4. **Age**
5. **Gender**
6. **Medications (diuretics/calcium channel blockers)**

Exercise 3-3: *Fill-in*

What are the six major types of urinary incontinence?

1. **Stress**
2. **Urge**
3. **Overflow**
4. **Reflex**
5. **Functional**
6. **Total incontinence**

Exercise 3-4: *Matching*

Match the type of urinary incontinence in Column A to its definition in Column B.

Column A		Column B
A. Stress	**D**	Inability to get to the toilet to urinate
B. Urge	**F**	Involuntary loss of urine that does not respond generally to treatment
C. Overflow	**A**	Loss of small amounts of urine when coughing, sneezing, or laughing
D. Functional	**E**	Involuntary loss of a moderate amount of urine usually without warning

Column A	Column B
E. Reflex	**B** Inability to stop urine flow long enough to reach toilet
F. Total incontinence	**C** Urinary retention associated with bladder overdistension

Exercise 3-5: *Fill-in*

Explain the significance of each of these tests as it relates to urinary incontinence.

1. Postvoid residual urine: **To detect urinary retention greater than 100 mL post void**
2. Urinalysis and urine culture/sensitivity: **To rule out a urinary tract infection**
3. Serum creatinine and BUN: **To assess function of the kidney**
4. Ultrasound of the bladder: **To detect abnormalities of the bladder and/or residual urine**

Exercise 3-6: *Select all that apply*

Which of the following interventions can control or eliminate Julia's incontinence?

☒ **Minimize delays in toileting**

☒ **Perform Kegel exercises**

☒ **Take prescribed diuretics in morning/mid-afternoon**

❏ Increase fluid intake at bedtime

☒ **Bladder retraining**

Exercise 3-7: *Multiple-choice question*

The nurse knows the best nursing diagnosis for Julia will be:

A. Pain—NO, although this is very possible, it is not the priority.

B. Activity intolerance—NO

C. Impaired urinary elimination—YES, this is the priority diagnosis.

D. Self-care deficit—NO

Exercise 3-8: *Fill-in*

The nurse suspects Simone of having a **urinary tract infection**.

Exercise 3-9: *Fill-in*

What presenting signs and symptoms indicate urinary tract infection for Simone?

1. **Frequent urination**
2. **Burning**
3. **Possible blood in urine**
4. **Unpleasant odor**
5. **Itching**

Exercise 3-10: *Fill-in*

The primary care provider has ordered a urinalysis and urine culture and sensitivity for Simone. Expected findings of the diagnostic testing will include: **may be positive for bacteria; sediment; white and red blood cells are noted and may be positive for leukocytes and nitrates**

Exercise 3-11: *Fill-in*

Name four side effects of Bactrim DS.
1. **Nausea**
2. **Rash/hives**
3. **Diarrhea**
4. **Difficulty breathing**

Exercise 3-12: *Select all that apply*

The nurse is explaining to Simone what she should expect with Macrobid. What should Simone expect to happen or expect to see with Macrobid?

☒ **Reddish/brown discoloration of urine**

☒ **Abdominal pain**

☒ **Photosensitivity**

☒ **Nausea/vomiting**

❑ Bulimia

Exercise 3-13: *Select all that apply*

The nurse is providing discharge teaching to Simone. What types of interventions will help Simone to decrease the risk of another urinary tract infection?

☒ **Urinate before and after intercourse**

☒ **Avoid wearing tight clothing**

☒ **Wipe the perineal area from front to back**

❑ Discourage fluid intake

☒ **Take all prescribed medications**

☒ **Avoid use of products containing perfumes**

Exercise 3-14: *Fill-in*

The primary care provider suspects a diagnosis of **urolithiasis.**

Exercise 3-15: *Select all that apply*

What can contribute to the formation of renal calculi?

☒ **Infection**

☒ **Prolonged acidic or alkaline urine**

☒ **Increased intake of calcium or oxalate-rich foods**

☒ **Decreased urine production**

❑ Decreased intake of calcium or oxalate-rich foods

Exercise 3-16: *Fill-in*
The primary care provider knows that the key symptom in urolithiasis is **pain**.

Exercise 3-17: *Multiple-choice question*
Grayson asks the primary care provider, "What is a cast?" The primary care provider replies:
A. Fatty deposits in the urine—NO, this does not describe a cast.
B. Glucose in the urine—NO, this does not describe a cast.
C. A type of tumor—NO, this does not describe a cast.
D. Cylinder particles made of white/red blood cells formed in the renal tubules—YES

Exercise 3-18: *Multiple-choice question*
What is the pathophysiologic reason for Grayson's nausea?
A. Gallbladder hematoma—NO, this is not the causative reason.
B. Dysphagia—NO, this is not the causative reason.
C. Severe pain—YES
D. Metabolic alkalosis—NO, this is not the causative reason.

Exercise 3-19: *Multiple-choice question*
Which of the following can contribute to the formation of renal calculi?
A. Hypothyroidism—NO, this is not identified as a cause.
B. Changes in urine pH—YES
C. Hypotension—NO, this is not identified as a cause.
D. Hypocalcemia—NO, this is not identified as a cause.

Exercise 3-20: *Multiple-choice question*
Which statement by Grayson lets the nurse know that he understands the purpose of a urine strainer?
A. "The urine strainer is to be used only when I have pain."—NO, it should be used all the time.
B. "The urine strainer is to strain all my urine for collection of the calculi."—YES
C. "The urine strainer is for my guests to use that visit me."—NO, this is a personal care item for the patient.
D. "The urine strainer is used to measure my urine output."—NO, it is not.

Exercise 3-21: *Fill-in*
Why does the presence of renal calculi put Grayson at risk for a UTI?
Calculi that are lodged in the ureter(s) or the bladder can obstruct the flow of urine. When urine flow is obstructed, bacteria are accumulated.

Exercise 3-22: *Multiple-choice question*

Which foods should Grayson have a low intake of?

  A. White potatoes/bananas—NO, this will not affect calculi formation.

  B. Peanut butter/milk—YES

  C. Legumes/fish—NO, this will not affect calculi formation.

  D. Fish/chicken—NO, this will not affect calculi formation.

Exercise 3-23: *Select all that apply*

What education is provided to Grayson before his discharge?

☒ **Follow prescribed dietary and medication regimens**

☒ **Encourage increased fluid intake**

☒ **Report signs and symptoms of pain**

☒ **Report the inability to void**

❑ Hematuria is a normal finding

Exercise 3-24: *Fill-in*

Based on Kimberly's signs/symptoms and metabolic results, the primary care provider is concerned about what pathophysiological process? **Acute renal failure.**

Exercise 3-25: *Multiple-choice question*

According to the metabolic results, what two lab values reflect the ability of the kidney to excrete waste?

  A. Sodium and chloride —NO

  B. Potassium and BUN—NO

  C. BUN and creatinine—YES

  D. Creatinine and sodium—NO

Exercise 3-26: *Multiple-choice question*

What acid–base balance process is occurring?

  A. Respiratory acidosis—NO

  B. Metabolic acidosis—YES

  C. Respiratory alkalosis—NO

  D. Metabolic alkalosis—NO

Exercise 3-27: *Fill-in*

Why is this acid–base process occurring?

The kidney is unable to secrete the excess hydrogen ions and conserve the bicarbonate, the kidney's buffering substance. Acidosis also occurs when the blood pH falls below 7.35.

Exercise 3-28: *Fill-in*

The primary care provider is also concerned that Kimberly's potassium level is 5.9 mEq/L. What is the pathophysiological process that is causing the elevation?

As the hydrogen ions increase, intracellular potassium (K+) moves to the extracellular fluid and the serum K+ level rises.

Exercise 3-29: *Multiple-choice question*

An elevated potassium level poses what immediate danger to Kimberly?

A. Disrupts the heart's conduction system—YES

B. Disrupts the lungs' exchange of air—NO

C. Disrupts the gastrointestinal system—NO

D. Disrupts the integumentary system—NO

Exercise 3-30: *Fill-in*

The urinalysis shows the presence of glucose and protein in the urine. What does this mean?

Glucose found in the urine would indicate the kidneys are not able to reabsorb the glucose; however, glucose found in the urine could also be an indication for diabetes.

Exercise 3-31: *Multiple-choice question*

The results of the urinalysis indicate the presence of casts. What damage do casts cause to the kidneys?

A. Damage to the urethra—NO

B. Damage to the tubules—YES

C. Damage to the bladder—NO

D. Damage to the anal orifice—NO

Exercise 3-32: *Select all that apply*

What urinalysis results indicate acute renal failure?

☒ **Protein**

☒ **Cells**

☒ **Casts**

❑ Specific gravity

❑ pH

❑ Glucose

Exercise 3-33: *Fill-in*

What is the purpose of diuresis in treating acute kidney failure?

Diuresis reduces the blood volume.

Exercise 3-34: *Fill-in*

Why is protein restricted in Kimberly's diet?

The kidneys are damaged and protein is abnormally filtered in the kidneys causing further damage to the glomeruli. When you decrease protein consumption, it will hopefully reduce further damage to the kidneys.

Exercise 3-35: *Fill-in*

What is renal dialysis?

Renal dialysis filters the waste products from the blood that cannot be filtered by the kidneys because the kidneys are damaged.

Exercise 3-36: *Fill-in*

What is hemodialysis?

Hemodialysis is when blood is pumped from the body to a filter where it is puri-fied and returned to the body.

What is peritoneal dialysis?

Peritoneal dialysis is when the body's peritoneal membrane is used as a filter. Fluid is drained in and out of the abdomen using a dialysate solution in pre-scribed concentrations.

Exercise 3-37: *Fill-in*

What is chronic renal failure?

A slow, progressive renal disorder related to kidney nephron loss. Chronic renal failure can occur over months or years and ultimately will lead to end-stage renal disease.

Exercise 3-38: *Fill-in*

Explain the five stages of chronic renal failure.

Stage I: **Minimal kidney damage with normal or relatively high glomerular filtra-tion rate (GFR) ($\supset$ 90 mL/min/1.73 m^2)**

Stage II: **Mild kidney damage with GFR (60–89 mL/min/1.73 m^2)**

Stage III: **Moderate reduction in GFR (30–59 mL/min/1.73 m^2)**

Stage IV: **Severe reduction in GFR (15–29 mL/min/1.73 m^2). Preparation for renal replacement therapy**

Stage V: **Established kidney failure (GFR $\subset$ 15 mL/min/1.73 m^2). Permanent renal replacement therapy or end-stage renal disease**

Exercise 3-39: *Select all that apply*

What are some symptoms of chronic renal disease?

☒ **Shortness of breath**

☒ **Fatigue or weakness**

☐ Increase in appetite

☒ **Nausea/vomiting**

☐ Urine output greater than 400 mL/day

Exercise 3-40: *Select all that apply*

What risk factors for chronic renal failure does Ethan present with?

☒ **Diabetes mellitus**

☒ **Hypertension**

❑ Drug toxicity

❑ Renal tuberculosis

❑ Congenital disorder

Exercise 3-41: *Multiple-choice question*

Ethan's blood glucose is within an acceptable range. His urinalysis was positive for blood and protein. What complication of diabetes might be occurring?

A. Hepatorenal syndrome—NO

B. Chronic renal failure related to diabetic nephropathy—YES

C. Acute renal failure related to urolithiasis—NO

D. Scleroderma—NO

Exercise 3-42: *Multiple-choice question*

What is generally the first sign of renal dysfunction in a diabetic patient?

A. Proteinuria—YES

B. Hyperkalemia—NO

C. Hyperparathyroidism—NO

D. Wilms's tumor—NO, this usually occurs in children.

Exercise 3-43: *Select all that apply*

What are some acute complications that may occur during Ethan's treatment?

☒ **Muscle cramps**

☒ **Angina**

☒ **Hypotension**

☒ **Arrhythmias**

☒ **Cardiac arrest**

❑ Bowel perforation

Exercise 3-44: *Fill-in*

Why must the nurse assess the graft for a thrill and bruit?

Absence of a thrill and bruit at a venous access site may indicate a blood clot that may require immediate surgical intervention.

Exercise 3-45: *Fill-in*

What are the two most common complications of a dialysis graft access?

1. **Thrombosis**

2. **Infection**

Exercise 3-46: *Select all that apply*

What is included in the aftercare by the nurse?

☒ **Monitor vascular access site for bleeding**

❏ Auscultate the thrill and palpate the bruit

☒ **Auscultate the bruit and palpate the thrill**

☒ **Vascular access site only used for treatment**

☒ **How to apply a dressing to graft site if bleeding occurs**

Exercise 3-47: *Multiple-choice question*

Ethan is being prepared for discharge to home. The nurse knows that Ethan needs further discharge instructions with this statement:

A. "I will keep my graft site clean and dry."—NO, this is something he should do.

B. "I will notify the primary care provider if I have swelling, redness, or drainage at my graft site."—NO, this is something he should do.

C. **"I can take my blood pressure in the same arm as my graft site."—YES, blood pressures should be done in the opposite arm.**

D. "I must avoid excessive pressure on my graft arm site."—NO, this is something he should do.

4

Nursing Care of the Patient With Gastrointestinal Disease

Karen K. Gittings

Unfolding Case Study #21 ▓ Craig

Craig is a 40-year-old male in good health, with a medical/surgical history of only renal calculi and an appendectomy. Recently, he has been experiencing a gnawing, burning pain in his mid-epigastric region. The pain is relieved by antacids or food. Craig has not sought medical attention prior to this point in time. This morning he noticed that his stool is a darker black color. At the urging of his wife, he has made an appointment with his primary care provider (PCP). The nurse has documented his chief complaint and reviewed his past medical history. His psychosocial history includes occasional alcohol use on the weekends, no smoking, and a high stress job in a small company. Recently, Craig has been taking ibuprofen 400 mg orally (PO) three times a day for a twisted ankle sustained while doing yard work.

Exercise 4-1: *Fill-in*
The nurse is aware that Craig's signs and symptoms are consistent with the clinical manifestations associated with: _____.

Exercise 4-2: *Select all that apply*
Identify factors that can cause and/or contribute to gastrointestinal ulceration (peptic ulcer disease):

- ❑ *Helicobacter pylori*
- ❑ Caffeinated beverages
- ❑ Milk ingestion
- ❑ High-protein diets
- ❑ Excessive smoking

(e) **eResource 4-1:** To learn more about factors that cause and/or contribute to gastrointestinal ulceration, go to Medscape: [Pathway: www.medscape .org → Under the tab "Reference," select "References & Tools" → enter "peptic ulcer disease" into the search field → select "overview" → select "Etiology" and review content]

Answers to this chapter begin on page 145.

Exercise 4-3: *Fill-in*

Identify Craig's risk factors for peptic ulcer disease and the rationale for how they place him at risk:

1. _____

2. _____

3. _____

4. _____

eResource 4-2: Consult Epocrates Online for detailed information related to Craig's risk factors associated with peptic ulcer disease: [Pathway: https://online.epocrates.com → select "Diseases" → enter "peptic ulcer disease" in the search field → under "Diagnosis" select "Risk Factors" and review content]

Craig's physician reviews his presenting signs and symptoms. His physical assessment of Craig reveals epigastric tenderness with palpation. A fecal occult blood test is done and the results are positive for blood in the stool, but the physician explains that a false-positive can occur with Hemoccult II testing. The physician explains that Craig likely has peptic ulcer disease with possible recent bleeding from the ulcerative site.

eResource 4-3: To learn more about interpretation of findings, consult Merck Manual: [Pathway: www.merckmanuals.com → select "The Merck Manual of Diagnosis and Therapy" → enter "GI Bleeding" into the search field in the upper right corner → select "Overview of GI Bleeding" → select "Interpretation of findings"]

eResource 4-4: Craig wants to know how he got the peptic ulcer in the first place. To help Craig understand this, the physician shows him a short video: *How a Peptic Ulcer Develops*: http://youtu.be/4bXZRgJ-1fk

Blood work is drawn for a complete blood count (CBC) and basic metabolic panel (BMP).

Exercise 4-4: *Select all that apply*

Identify clinical manifestations associated with peptic ulcer disease:

❑ Diffuse abdominal tenderness

❑ Pyrosis

❑ Melena

❑ Frequent vomiting

❑ Sour eructation

eResource 4-5: Consult Medscape for more information related to clinical manifestations/presentation of peptic ulcer disease: [Pathway: www.medscape.org → Under the tab "Reference," select "References & Tools" → enter "peptic ulcer disease" into the search field → select "Presentation"→ select "History" and "Physical Examination" and review

Answers to this chapter begin on page 145.

content; be sure to click on "Multimedia Library" in this section to review the related images]

Exercise 4-5: *Matching*

Match the type of ulcer in Column A with its common characteristics in Column B. Answers in Column A can be used more than once.

Column A	Column B
A. Duodenal ulcer	_____ 80% of ulcers are this type
B. Gastric ulcer	_____ Usually occurs in people older than 50 years
	_____ Associated with hypersecretion of hydrochloric acid (HCl)
	_____ Pain occurs 2 to 3 hours after meal
	_____ Ingestion of food does not help pain
	_____ Hematemesis more common

eResource 4-6: To learn more about gastrointestinal bleeding, listen to Merck Medicus's podcast: *Gastrointestinal Bleeding*: http://goo.gl/LFjf3

Exercise 4-6: *True or false*

Identify whether the following statements about Hemoccult II stool testing for occult blood are true or false:

_____ 1. Aspirin and nonsteroidal anti-inflammatory drugs (NSAIDs) may cause a false-positive result.

_____ 2. Turnips and horseradish should be avoided for 72 hours prior to testing because they may cause a false-positive result.

_____ 3. Vitamin C supplements may cause a false-positive result.

_____ 4. Red meat may cause a false-positive result if ingested within 72 hours prior to testing.

Exercise 4-7: *Fill-in*

Identify three nursing diagnoses for the patient with peptic ulcer disease:

1. _____

2. _____

3. _____

eResource 4-7: For more information regarding nursing diagnoses, review the following:

- Video on *How to Write a Nursing Diagnosis*: http://youtu.be/JyAaQ5hILSs
- The NANDA Nursing Diagnosis List: http://goo.gl/1ryZg

Craig is scheduled for an endoscopy on the following day. The nurse gives him pre-procedure instructions and informs him to arrive at the hospital at 8:00 a.m. so that he can register and be prepped before the scheduled time of the procedure.

Answers to this chapter begin on page 145.

Exercise 4-8: *Multiple-choice question*

After educating Craig on the endoscopy procedure and pre-procedure instructions, the nurse determines that he understands the information when he states:

    A. "I will have to stay in the hospital overnight after this procedure."

    B. "I will have to have anesthesia in the operating room during the procedure."

    C. "I will be sedated so they can pass a scope down into my stomach and intestine."

    D. "I will have to have my bowels cleaned out prior to this procedure."

 eResource 4-8: Consult Medscape for more information related to the endoscopy: [Pathway: www.medscape.org → Under the tab "Reference," select "References & Tools" → enter "Endoscopy" into the search field → select "Capsule Endoscopy" and review content; be sure to click on "Multimedia Library" in this section to review the related images]

Exercise 4-9: *Multiple-choice question*

As Craig asks further questions about the endoscopy, the nurse determines that he needs further instruction when he states:

    A. "Since this procedure only takes about 30 minutes, I will be able to drive myself home afterward."

    B. "I will be sure not to eat or drink anything after midnight tonight."

    C. "They will spray the back of my throat so I don't gag on the tube."

    D. "The doctor will be able to see if I have an ulcer and treat any bleeding."

After the endoscopy is completed and Craig has recovered from the conscious sedation, the physician arrives to discuss his findings. A small, nonbleeding ulcer was located in the duodenum. A biopsy of the mucosa has been sent to the lab for testing, but the appearance is suggestive of infection with *H. pylori*. The physician discusses the medication that will be used to treat the *H. pylori* and duodenal ulcer.

Exercise 4-10: *Matching*

Match the medication used to treat peptic ulcer disease and *H. pylori* infection in Column A with its action in Column B.

Column A	Column B
A. amoxicillin (Amoxil)	_____ Decreases gastric acid secretion by slowing H^+, K^+-ATPase pump
B. metronidazole (Flagyl)	_____ Bactericidal antibiotic that eradicates *H. pylori*
C. bismuth subsalicylate (Pepto-Bismol)	_____ Synthetic antibacterial and anti-protozoal agent that eradicates *H. pylori*
D. omeprazole (Prilosec)	_____ Suppresses *H. pylori* and assists with healing of mucosal ulcers

Answers to this chapter begin on page 145.

eResource 4-9: Consult Epocrates on your mobile device to review safety and monitoring guidelines that you would want to share with Craig: [Pathway: Epocrates → select "amoxicillin" → select "Safety/Monitoring." Also review Contraindications/Cautions as well as Adverse Reactions. Repeat this with the other drugs]

Craig is ready for discharge home. He is given prescriptions for clarithromycin 500 mg PO twice a day (bid), amoxicillin 1000 mg PO bid, and omeprazole 20 mg PO daily. He is instructed to complete his 14-day course of antibiotics, even if he is feeling better and without symptoms. He will need to take his proton pump inhibitor (PPI) for at least 4 weeks. The nurse gives further instructions about his diet and follow-up care.

eResource 4-10: To learn more about PPIs, consult the Merck Manual: [Pathway: www.merckmanuals.com → select "The Merck Manual of Diagnosis and Therapy" → enter "peptic ulcer disease" into the search field in the upper right corner → select "Drug Treatment of Gastric Acidity" and review content]

Exercise 4-11: *Select all that apply*
Identify recommended dietary changes for patients with peptic ulcer disease:
- ❑ Replace coffee with decaffeinated coffee
- ❑ Avoid extreme temperatures in food and drinks
- ❑ Eat three regular meals per day
- ❑ Increase milk intake
- ❑ Avoid alcohol

eResource 4-11: Download AHRQ's Electronic Preventive Services Selector (ePSS) onto your mobile device or computer (http://epss.ahrq .gov/PDA/index.jsp) and enter Craig's personal data to identify clinical preventive services that are appropriate for him.

Unfolding Case Study #22 ▨ Chad

Chad is a 28-year-old male who has been in good health. Today he presents to the emergency department (ED) with a complaint of abdominal pain and nausea. He has no past medical or surgical history. His vital signs are as follows: temperature 100.4°F, pulse 108 beats/min, respirations 26 breaths/min, and blood pressure 146/84. Chad is sent for a computed tomographic (CT) scan of the abdomen, after which he is diagnosed with appendicitis.

eResource 4-12: To learn more about CT scanning, go to Medscape: [Pathway: www.medscape.org → Under the tab "Reference," select "References & Tools" → enter "Appendicitis Workup" into the search field → select "CT Scanning"→ select "History" and "Physical Examination" and review content; be sure to click on "Imaging of Appendicitis" in this section to review the related images]

Exercise 4-12: *Multiple-choice question*

In the United States, appendicitis is the most common cause of an acute abdomen requiring surgery. This is related to the fact that the appendix:

    A. is prone to obstruction leading to inflammation, edema, and infection.

    B. has no useful function in the body.

    C. is easily inflamed by eating hot, spicy foods.

    D. is easily traumatized during contact sports and vehicular accidents.

Exercise 4-13: *Select all that apply*

Identify clinical manifestations exhibited by patients with acute appendicitis:

    ❑ Abdominal pain

    ❑ Low-grade fever

    ❑ Diarrhea

    ❑ Bloody stools

    ❑ Nausea with/without vomiting

    ❑ Rovsing's sign

    ❑ Rebound tenderness

Exercise 4-14: *Fill-in*

Briefly explain/describe the abdominal pain associated with appendicitis, including whether it is diffuse or localized.

_____

_____

_____

 eResource 4-13: Consult Epocrates Online for detailed information related to Appendicitis: [Pathway: https://online.epocrates.com → select "Diseases" → enter "appendicitis" in the search field → under "Diagnosis" select "History & Exam" and review "Key Diagnostic Factors"]

Answers to this chapter begin on page 145.

Exercise 4-15: *Hot spot*

Mark the area where you would elicit pain at McBurney's point in patients with appendicitis:

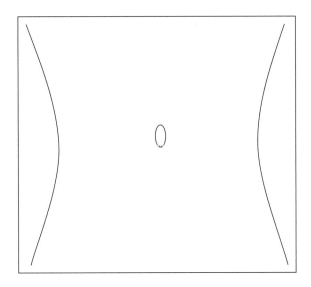

Blood work is sent for a CBC and BMP. A #20-gauge intravenous (IV) catheter is inserted in the left arm. An IV solution of 0.9% saline (NaCl) is started infusing at 75 mL/hr. The surgeon visits Chad in the ED and informed consent is obtained for an appendectomy.

 eResource 4-14: To provide an informed consent from Chad, the surgeon reviews the appendectomy procedure, *3D Medical Animation-Laparoscopic Appendectomy Surgery*: http://goo.gl/cYgNq

Chad will be taken to surgery within the next 2 hours.

Exercise 4-16: *Fill-in*

Identify the tonicity of the following IV solutions:

1. 0.9% NaCl _____

2. D5NS _____

3. 0.45% NaCl _____

4. Lactated Ringer's _____

5. 3% NaCl _____

6. D5 0.45% NaCl _____

Exercise 4-17: *Fill-in*

Briefly explain the role of the physician and the nurse in obtaining informed consent.

_____

_____

After surgery is complete, Chad is transferred to the recovery room and from there to a bed in the surgical unit. The surgeon was unable to perform the surgery laparoscopically, so an open appendectomy was performed.

Physician orders include:

- Nothing by mouth (NPO)
- IV of Lactated Ringer's at 100 mL/hr
- Intake and output (I&O) every 8 hours
- Piperacillin/tazobactam (Zosyn) 3.375 g IV every 6 hours
- Morphine 4 mg IV every 2 hours as needed (PRN) for severe pain
- Sequential compression devices while in bed
- Incentive spirometry 10 breaths every 1 to 2 hours

After getting Chad settled into his new room, the nurse completes her assessment. Chad reports that his pain level is 8 out of 10 in the area of his incision.

Exercise 4-18: *Calculation*

Order: Morphine 4 mg IV every 2 hours PRN for severe pain.

If the morphine is supplied 10 mg per 2 mL, calculate how much morphine (in mL) you would administer? _____

e **eResource 4-15:** Use MedCalc to verify your answer: [Pathway: www .medcalc.com → select "Fluids/Electrolytes" → select "IV Rate" and enter information into fields]

Exercise 4-19: *Fill-in*

Identify three potential complications that can occur postoperatively in the patient with appendicitis:

1. _____

2. _____

3. _____

e **eResource 4-16:** Consult Medscape for more information related to postoperative considerations for an Open Appendectomy: [Pathway: www.medscape.org → Under the tab "Reference," select "References & Tools" → enter "Appendectomy" into the search field → select "Open Appendectomy"→ select "Postoperative Follow-up" and review content; be sure to click on "Multimedia Library" in this section to review the related images]

e **eResource 4-17:** To view a brief video clip demonstrating an open appendectomy, go to: http://goo.gl/WwPKp

Exercise 4-20: *Fill-in*

Identify three nursing diagnoses for the patient with appendicitis:

1. _____

2. _____

3. _____

 eResource 4-18: For more information regarding nursing diagnoses, refer to the NANDA Nursing Diagnosis List: http://goo.gl/1ryZg

Exercise 4-21: *Matching*

Match the nursing intervention in Column A with its intended effect/purpose in Column B.

Column A	Column B
A. Diaphragmatic breathing	_____ Minimizes the risk of postoperative wound infection
B. Leg exercises	_____ Maintains a comfort level that allows the patient to participate in care
C. Pain control	_____ Promotes optimal lung expansion and blood oxygenation
D. Splint the incision	_____ Improves circulation and prevents venous stasis
E. Good hand washing	_____ Minimizes pressure and pain when coughing

Exercise 4-22: *True or false*

Identify whether the following statements about postoperative nursing interventions are true or false:

_____ 1. Incentive spirometry is a device that measures and provides feedback on the effectiveness of the patient's breathing.

_____ 2. Sequential compression devices are effective in maintaining the patient's muscle strength while bedridden.

_____ 3. Wound assessment and dressing changes are important for early identification of wound infection.

On his second day postoperatively, Chad is recovering well. He is eating and tolerating a regular diet. He is ambulating in the hallway. Percocet is effective in controlling his pain. It is anticipated that Chad will be discharged home in the morning.

 eResource 4-19: Consult Epocrates on your mobile device to review safety and monitoring guidelines that you would want to share with Chad: [Pathway: Epocrates → select "Percocet" → select "Safety/ Monitoring." Also review Contraindications/Cautions as well as Adverse Reactions]

Answers to this chapter begin on page 145.

Exercise 4-23: *Multiple-choice question*

After educating Chad on his discharge instructions, the nurse determines that he understands the information when he states:

 A. "I should call the physician if I feel nauseated."
 B. "I should double my preoperative caloric intake while I am still healing."
 C. "I need to avoid heavy lifting until directed by my physician."
 D. "I should take a bath daily to soak my abdominal incision."

 eResource 4-20: Consult Epocrates Online for detailed information related to discharge instructions to Chad following the appendectomy: [Pathway: https://online.epocrates.com → select "Diseases" → enter "appendicitis" in the search field → select "acute appendicitis" → under "Follow-Up" select "Overview" and "Complications"]

Unfolding Case Study #23 ▬ Stephanie

Stephanie is a 58-year-old female who presents to the ED with complaints of abdominal pain, nausea, and vomiting. On physical assessment, abdominal distension is noted. The physician orders an IV line inserted and 0.9% NaCl started at 75 mL/hr. Blood work is sent for a CBC, complete metabolic panel (CMP), amylase, and lipase. An abdominal x-ray and CT scan are also ordered. The laboratory results are noted in Table 4-1:

Table 4-1: Laboratory Results

Laboratory Test	Results
Glucose	110 mg/dL
Sodium	147 mEq/L
Chloride	110 mEq/L
Potassium	3.5 mEq/L
BUN	30 mg/dL
Creatinine	1.8 mg/dL
Osmolality	315 mOsm/kg water
Red blood cells (RBCs)	4.8×10^{12}/L
Hemoglobin (Hgb)	14.4 g/dL
Hematocrit (Hct)	37%
White blood cells (WBCs)	14,500/mm^3
Amylase	150 U/L
Lipase	90 U/L

Answers to this chapter begin on page 145.

Exercise 4-24: *Fill-in*

Identify which of Stephanie's laboratory values are abnormal and whether it is high or low:

1. _____

2. _____

3. _____

4. _____

5. _____

6. _____

> **eResource 4-21:** Consult Stedman's Laboratory Reference Range Values: http://goo.gl/tXI3a

Exercise 4-25: *Fill-in*

Provide a brief explanation of why the blood results may be abnormal.

_____

_____

_____

Stephanie's abdominal x-ray and CT scan show an abnormal amount of gas and fluid in the small intestine. She is diagnosed with a small bowel obstruction. A surgeon is consulted to evaluate whether Stephanie needs surgery.

> **eResource 4-22:** To learn more about small bowel obstruction, go to Medscape: [Pathway: www.medscape.org → Under the tab "Reference," select "References & Tools" → enter "small bowel obstruction" into the search field → select "Overview" and review content; be sure to view multimedia library]

The nurse completes an admission history. Stephanie has a medical history of anxiety and hypertension. She has a surgical history of a cholecystectomy and two cesarean births.

Exercise 4-26: *Fill-in*

Identify the two types of intestinal obstructions with a brief description and example of both:

1. _____

2. _____

Exercise 4-27: *Matching*

Match the cause of intestinal obstruction in Column A with its description in Column B.

Column A	Column B
A. Adhesions	_____ Bowel twists and turns on itself
B. Intussusception	_____ Bowel protrudes through a weakened abdominal muscle or wall
C. Volvulus	_____ One part of the bowel slips into another part
D. Hernia	_____ A tumor within the intestinal wall protrudes into the lumen
E. Tumor	_____ Bowel becomes adherent to scarred areas after abdominal surgery

Exercise 4-28: *Fill-in*

Identify Stephanie's risk factors for developing an intestinal obstruction with an explanation for why these put her at risk:

_____

_____

e **eResource 4-23:** Consult Epocrates Online for detailed information related to Stephanie's risk factors associated with small bowel obstruction: [Pathway: https://online.epocrates.com → select "Diseases" → enter "small bowel obstruction" in the search field → under "Diagnosis" select "Risk Factors" and review content]

Exercise 4-29: *Select all that apply*

Identify clinical manifestations exhibited by patients with small bowel obstructions:

- ❑ Crampy, wave-like abdominal pain
- ❑ Increased flatus
- ❑ Fecal vomiting
- ❑ Abdominal distension
- ❑ Dehydration
- ❑ Large, hardened bowel movements

e **eResource 4-24:** To learn more about the clinical presentation, go to Medscape: [Pathway: www.medscape.org → Under the tab "Reference," select "References & Tools" → enter "small bowel obstruction" into the search field → select "Presentation"→ review "History" and "Physical Examination"]

Stephanie is admitted to the surgical floor. She is ordered to be NPO. Her IV fluids of 0.9% NaCl are ordered to be increased to 125 mL/hr. She is to have a nasogastric (NG) tube inserted and placed to continuous low wall suction. The surgeon has informed Stephanie that he is going to see if the nasogastric suction will resolve her small bowel obstruction. The nurse prepares Stephanie for insertion of the NG tube.

Exercise 4-30: *Ordering*

Number in order the steps required for insertion of a NG tube:

_____ Explain the purpose of the tube and procedure for insertion.

_____ Lubricate the tube with water-soluble lubricant.

_____ Confirm the physician's order.

_____ Sit the patient upright in bed.

_____ Instruct the patient to lower head as tube reaches nasopharynx.

_____ Gather supplies.

_____ Confirm tube placement.

_____ Identify the patient.

_____ Instruct the patient to swallow as tube is advanced.

_____ Secure tube to nose.

_____ Measure from the tip of the nose to the earlobe to the xiphoid process.

_____ Apply clean gloves.

e **eResource 4-25:** To review the procedure of NG tube insertion, consult Medscape: [Pathway: www.medscape.org → Under the tab "Reference," select "References & Tools" → enter "NGT" into the search field → select "Nasogastric Tube"→ review content focusing on "Positioning," "Technique," and "Pearls"]

Exercise 4-31: *True or false*

Identify whether the following statements about assessing NG tube placement are true or false:

_____ 1. X-ray visualization of the tube tip is the most accurate method for verifying placement.

_____ 2. Air auscultation is a traditional method that has been shown to be a reliable indicator of tube placement.

_____ 3. Visual assessment of aspirate color is effective in ruling out respiratory placement.

_____ 4. Gastric pH measurements are affected by continuous tube feedings and proton pump inhibitors.

Stephanie has had a NG tube in place for 36 hours. She asks the nurse when it will be removed and when she will be able to have something to drink. Stephanie is scheduled for an abdominal x-ray this morning to evaluate the progress of the small bowel obstruction. The nurse answers Stephanie's questions and explains the importance of the follow-up abdominal x-ray.

Exercise 4-32: *Multiple-choice question*

Decompression of the bowel is successful in most cases, but surgery may be warranted if:

   A. The patient has had an NG tube for 12 hours.

   B. The NG tube is draining bile-colored contents.

   C. The patient is uncomfortable with the NG tube.

   D. The bowel is completely obstructed and causing necrosis.

Stephanie's abdominal x-ray shows clearing of the small bowel obstruction. The NG tube is discontinued, and she is started on a clear liquid diet. The nurse orders a clear liquid tray for lunch and asks Stephanie what she would like to drink until the tray arrives.

Exercise 4-33: *Fill-in*

Briefly explain/describe a clear liquid diet, including indications for use with Stephanie.

_____

_____

_____

_____

Exercise 4-34: *Select all that apply*

Identify foods/liquids permitted with a clear liquid diet:

   ❑ Ginger ale

   ❑ Popsicles

   ❑ Orange juice

   ❑ Milk

   ❑ Clear broth

eResource 4-26: For more information regarding a clear liquid diet, refer to:
   ■ Mayo Clinic's Clear Liquid Diet overview: http://goo.gl/gjAz
   ■ MedlinePlus's Diet-clear liquid: http://goo.gl/6JLW3

Stephanie continues to do well. She is tolerating clear liquids without nausea or vomiting. She has active bowel sounds in four quadrants and is passing flatus. Stephanie is advanced to full liquid diet and discharge is planned for the following day.

Unfolding Case Study #24 ▨ John

John is a 67-year-old male who is at his physician's office for his 6-month visit. His medical history includes hypertension, benign prostatic hyperplasia, and polyps. He was a one pack per day (PPD) smoker until he quit 2 years ago. Since quitting smoking, John's weight has increased so that he is now obese, with minimal daily physical activity. John reports to the nurse that he has been feeling more tired

Answers to this chapter begin on page 145.

lately and that he is having problems with constipation. He also reports that he has noticed some blood in his stools. The physician listens to John's chief complaint, reviews his past medical history, and then takes a family history.

 eResource 4-27: Consult AHRQ's Electronic Preventive Services Selector (ePSS) on your mobile device or computer (http://epss.ahrq.gov/PDA/index.jsp) and enter John's personal data to identify clinical preventive services that are appropriate for him.

It is discovered that John has a history of colon cancer in his immediate family. On assessment, the physician notes abdominal distension and a fecal occult blood test is positive for blood. Laboratory tests are ordered and John is scheduled for a colonoscopy in 2 days.

Exercise 4-35: *Fill-in*
Identify John's risk factors for colorectal cancer:

1. _____

2. _____

3. _____

4. _____

5. _____

 eResource 4-28: To learn more about risk factors for colon cancer, view the American Cancer Society's video, *Colon Cancer Risk Factors: What You Need to Know*: http://youtu.be/5w9dR1X2wOE

Exercise 4-36: *Select all that apply*
Identify additional risk factors for colorectal cancer:

❑ Benign prostatic hyperplasia
❑ High-fat, high-protein, low-fiber diet
❑ Hypertension
❑ History of heavy alcohol use
❑ History of inflammatory bowel disease

 eResource 4-29: Consult Epocrates Online for more detailed information related to John's risk factors for colon cancer: [Pathway: https://online .epocrates.com → select "Diseases" → enter "colon cancer" in the search field → under "Diagnosis" select "Risk Factors" and review content]

Exercise 4-37: *Fill-in*
The most common presenting symptom of colorectal cancer is _____
and the second most common is _____.

Answers to this chapter begin on page 145.

eResource 4-30: Consult Epocrates Online for more detailed information about key diagnostic factors: [Pathway: https://online.epocrates.com → select "Diseases" → enter "colon cancer" in the search field → under "Diagnosis" select "History & Exam" and review content]

Exercise 4-38: *Matching*

Match the location of the lesion or tumor in Column A with its commonly associated symptoms in Column B. Answers in Column A can be used more than once.

Column A	Column B
A. Right-sided lesions	_____ Cramping pain
B. Left-sided lesions	_____ Ineffective, painful straining at stool
C. Rectal lesions	_____ Melena
	_____ Abdominal distension
	_____ Narrow stools
	_____ Feeling of incomplete evacuation after bowel movement

Before John leaves the physician's office, he is given instructions on how to prepare for the colonoscopy.

 eResource 4-31: John also views a MedlinePlus video, which provides an overview of the colonoscopy procedure: http://goo.gl/wOm8n

He is also given an order for laboratory tests to be drawn, including a CBC, BMP, ferritin level, and carcinoembryonic antigen (CEA).

Exercise 4-39: *Multiple-choice question*

Lavage solutions, such as GoLYTELY, are effective in cleansing the bowel for optimal visualization, but side effects include:

    A. Nausea, vomiting, and fluid overload
    B. Bloating, constipation, and painful straining at stools
    C. Nausea, cramps, and constipation
    D. Cramps, abdominal fullness, and fluid/electrolyte imbalances

Exercise 4-40: *Fill-in*

Briefly explain how CEA is used as a prognostic predictor of cancer and the effectiveness of treatment.

_____

_____

_____

eResource 4-32: To learn more about the CEA test, visit Lab Tests Online: http://goo.gl/Hh3Ge

John's colonoscopy is completed without problem.

 eResource 4-33: To learn more about the procedure and postprocedure care, consult Medscape: [Pathway: www.medscape.org → Under the tab "Reference," select "References & Tools" → enter "Colonoscopy" into the search field → review content focusing on "Post-Procedure"]

The gastroenterologist talks to John's wife about his findings and plans to come back to see John when he is fully recovered, awake, and alert. He explains that John will stay in the outpatient recovery room until he is fully recovered and stable, at which point he will be discharged home.

Exercise 4-41: *Select all that apply*

Identify interventions used to monitor patients after colonoscopy to ensure a safe recovery:

- ❏ Monitor oxygen saturation
- ❏ Check vital signs hourly for 4 hours, then every 4 hours
- ❏ Monitor for worsening abdominal pain or distension
- ❏ Monitor level of consciousness

After John is fully recovered, the doctor returns to discuss his findings. A tumor was located in the descending colon near the upper sigmoid area. John has been scheduled to see a general surgeon in 1 week and he is discharged home. John and his wife are visibly upset. The nurse talks with them before sending John home.

 eResource 4-34: To learn more about the six-step protocol for giving bad news, view *How Best to Deliver Bad News to Patients and Family:* http://youtu.be/ItC68Pdnpk4

Exercise 4-42: *Multiple-choice question*

When John states that he is scared that he is going to die, the nurse's best response is:

- A. "Don't worry; everything is going to be okay."
- B. "I know someone who had cancer; I can tell you their story."
- C. "It must be very frightening for you to have just received this diagnosis."
- D. "I can try to find someone to talk with you further."

 eResource 4-35: For a review of Therapeutic Communication, view
- ■ Therapeutic Communication in Psychiatric Nursing: http://goo.gl/UnCdX
- ■ List of Communication Techniques: http://goo.gl/LSgMJ

Answers to this chapter begin on page 145.

One week later, John has an appointment with his surgeon, who has already reviewed the results of John's colonoscopy. The surgeon further explains the diagnosis and the planned procedure, and John gives informed consent for surgery to be done. Surgery is scheduled for 1 week later. John is given preoperative instructions for diet, bowel cleansing, and a prescription for cephalexin (Keflex).

 eResource 4-36: To learn more about the procedure and informed consent:
- View the video, *Colectomy*: http://goo.gl/QT53Z
- Read *Informed Consent—Adults* from MedlinePlus: http://goo.gl/G79rW

Exercise 4-43: *Fill-in*

John is put on a diet high in calories, protein, and carbohydrates and low in residue after his appointment. Twenty-four hours before surgery, he is changed to a full liquid diet. Briefly explain the rationale behind these dietary orders.

_____

_____

_____

_____

Exercise 4-44: *Multiple-choice question*

When John asks why he needs to take an antibiotic the day before surgery, the nurse's best response is:

- A. "This is done prophylactically to prevent infection."
- B. "The cephalexin (Keflex) will reduce the bacteria in your intestines before surgery."
- C. "The tumor is already causing an infection in your body."
- D. "It is given the day before surgery to start your antibiotics early."

 eResource 4-37: The nurse provides additional patient teaching and gives John the *Patient Handbook for Colectomy*: http://goo.gl/U4YmV

Two weeks after his diagnosis, John is admitted to the hospital for a scheduled bowel resection and temporary colostomy. Preoperatively, he watched a video on colostomy care, and he met the Wound, Ostomy, and Continence (WOC) nurse that will be working with him postoperatively.

 eResource 4-38: Patient self-care teaching material: http://goo.gl/vfU88

Exercise 4-45: *Matching*

Match the colostomy site in Column A with its expected fecal output in Column B.

Column A	**Column B**
A. Ascending colostomy	_____ Unformed stool
B. Transverse colostomy	_____ Formed stool
C. Descending colostomy	_____ Fluid stool
D. Sigmoid colostomy	_____ Semi-formed stool

John's surgery is successfully completed, and he is transferred to a room on the surgical floor. The WOC nurse works with him every day to ensure that he understands how to care for his colostomy, where to obtain supplies, and dietary considerations related to the colostomy.

Exercise 4-46: *Select all that apply*

Identify foods that cause excessive gas and odor and should therefore be avoided:

- ❑ Asparagus
- ❑ Milk
- ❑ Eggs
- ❑ Beans
- ❑ Tomatoes
- ❑ Cabbage

Exercise 4-47: *True or false*

Identify whether the following statements about colostomy care are true or false:

_____ 1. A stoma that is beefy red or pink in color is healthy and indicates good circulation.

_____ 2. The colostomy should begin functioning within 12 hours of surgery.

_____ 3. Colostomy appliances should be changed every 24 hours to avoid leakage.

_____ 4. Empty the colostomy appliance when it is one-third full to prevent the appliance from separating from the skin.

John is soon discharged home with follow-up appointments with his surgeon, an oncologist, and the WOC nurse. He and his wife were very engaged during teaching sessions, and they have both become skilled at colostomy care.

Answers to this chapter begin on page 145.

Unfolding Case Study #25 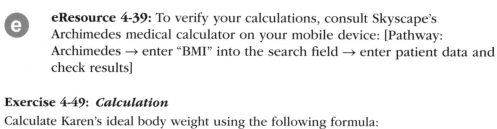 Karen

Karen is a 49-year-old female who has come to her primary care provider (PCP) to discuss her weight problems. At 5 feet 5 inches and 295 pounds, Karen is considered morbidly obese. She has a history of being up and down on her weight since her early 20s. Her weight increases primarily when she is in school and then decreases when she is able to resume exercising and increase her activity level. Twice in her life, Karen has dieted down to her ideal body weight. Karen was diagnosed with type 2 diabetes and hypertension within the past 5 years. She recognizes the risks associated with her obesity and the importance of regaining a healthier weight, but she is struggling to maintain a healthy weight loss diet and increase her exercise. Karen is seeking the advice of the PCP.

Exercise 4-48: *Calculation*
Calculate Karen's body mass index (BMI) using the following formula:

BMI = 703 × weight in pounds/(height in inches)^2

---

e   **eResource 4-39:** To verify your calculations, consult Skyscape's Archimedes medical calculator on your mobile device: [Pathway: Archimedes → enter "BMI" into the search field → enter patient data and check results]

Exercise 4-49: *Calculation*
Calculate Karen's ideal body weight using the following formula:

❏ Allow 100 pounds for 5 feet of height

❏ Add 5 pounds for each additional inch over 5 feet

❏ Subtract 10% for small frames; add 10% for large frames

---

e   **eResource 4-40:** To verify your calculations, consult Skyscape's Archimedes medical calculator on your mobile device: [Pathway: Archimedes → enter "Ideal Body Weight" into the search field → enter patient data and check results]

Exercise 4-50: *Select all that apply*
Identify health risks associated with morbid obesity:
      ❏ Chronic obstructive pulmonary disease
      ❏ Diabetes
      ❏ Heart disease
      ❏ Gallbladder disease
      ❏ Urinary tract infections
      ❏ Sleep apnea

Answers to this chapter begin on page 145.

eResource 4-41: The primary care provider knows that obesity is a problem among many Americans and recalls watching *The Obesity Epidemic*, a video from the CDC: http://goo.gl/NbZsc

Karen and her PCP discuss her current eating and activity patterns in order to develop a plan for weight loss. Karen states that she eats out a lot, especially fast food. At home, she primarily eats soup, frozen dinners, or canned foods, like beef stew. She is active 2 days a week when she is in the hospital with nursing students, but other days, she is primarily working at a desk. She is involved in no other form of exercise. Karen and her PCP discuss dietary therapy, physical activity, behavior modification, and the new weight loss medication, Qsymia.

Exercise 4-51: *True or false*
Identify whether the following statements about lifestyle and food intake are true or false:

_____ 1. People who regularly skip breakfast are less likely to be obese.
_____ 2. Eating meals out is associated with a lower food intake.
_____ 3. The faster food is eaten, the greater the food intake.
_____ 4. The greater the variety of food, the more kilocalories consumed.

Exercise 4-52: *Fill-in*
A weight loss diet should be reduced in total kilocalories, but also meet the following requirements:
1. Carbohydrates _____ % of kilocalories
2. Fat _____ % of kilocalories
3. Protein _____ % of kilocalories
4. _____ % of kilocalories open to negotiation
5. Fiber _____ grams

Exercise 4-53: *Multiple-choice question*
After discussing exercise for weight loss, the PCP determines that Karen needs further instruction when she states:

A. "I should begin with 30 to 45 minutes of exercise 3 to 5 days per week."
B. "I need to drink water before, during, and after exercise, especially in hot weather."
C. "In order to maintain weight loss, I will have to continue exercising even after reaching my goal."
D. "The only way to continue to lose weight is by running."

Answers to this chapter begin on page 145.

Exercise 4-54: *Fill-in*

Identify five behavior modification techniques recommended to facilitate weight loss:

1. _____

2. _____

3. _____

4. _____

5. _____

(e) eResource 4-42: To learn more about obesity treatment and management, go to Medscape: [Pathway: www.medscape.org → Under the tab "Reference," select "References & Tools" → enter "obesity" into the search field → select "Obesity," → select "Treatment" and review content]

Exercise 4-55: *Fill-in*

Two potential side effects associated with the new weight loss medication Qsymia are _____ and _____.

After 6 months of dieting, exercise, behavior modification, and pharmacotherapy with Qsymia, Karen has seen no significant reduction in her weight. Her PCP has referred her to a bariatric surgeon. She has completed her counseling, education, and evaluation by the multidisciplinary health care team and has been cleared for surgery.

Exercise 4-56: *Fill-in*

Bariatric surgeries aid in weight loss through _____, _____, or both.

Exercise 4-57: *True or false*

Identify whether the following statements about selection criteria for bariatric surgery are true or false:

_____ 1. To be eligible for bariatric surgery, all patients must have a BMI greater than 40 kg/m².

_____ 2. Patients are expected to adhere to postoperative care, medical management, and follow-up visits after bariatric surgery.

_____ 3. A patient will be excluded from surgery if he or she is unable to comprehend the risks, benefits, and lifestyle changes required.

_____ 4. Patients are not required to have a history of failed dieting or other nonsurgical attempts at weight loss prior to surgical intervention.

Exercise 4-58: *Select all that apply*

Identify common complications that can occur after bariatric surgery:

❑ Bleeding

❑ Leaking from anastomosis site

Answers to this chapter begin on page 145.

❑ Unstable blood sugars

❑ Dehydration

❑ Nausea

❑ Change in bowel function

 eResource 4-43: To learn more about the bariatric surgical procedure, go to Medscape: [Pathway: www.medscape.org → Under the tab "Reference," select "References & Tools" → enter "Bariatric surgery" into the search field → select "Bariatric surgery" → select "Treatment" and review content]

Karen has her bariatric surgery and is recovering postoperatively in a surgical unit. She had a Roux-en-Y gastric bypass, which is recommended for long-term weight loss. After having an upper gastrointestinal study to confirm no leaking from the anastomosis site, Karen is started on a post-gastric surgery diet.

Exercise 4-59: *Select all that apply*

Identify dietary guidelines for the patient post bariatric surgery:

❑ Eat 3 to 6 small meals per day

❑ Choose foods low in calories and nutrients

❑ Avoid drinking while eating

❑ Restrict total meal size to less than 1 cup

❑ Avoid concentrated sources of carbohydrates

❑ Finish eating meals even if feeling full

Exercise 4-60: *Multiple-choice question*

In order to avoid dumping syndrome, which sometimes occurs after gastric surgery, the nurse should teach the patient the following prevention strategies, with the exception of:

A. Meals should contain more dry items than liquid.

B. Fluid intake with meals is discouraged.

C. Remain in a low Fowler's position for 20 to 30 minutes after meals.

D. Decrease fat intake and increase intake of concentrated carbohydrates.

 eResource 4-44: To learn more about dumping syndrome, refer to
  ▪ Mayo Clinic's tip sheet, Dumping Syndrome: http://goo.gl/k3AY0
  ▪ Dumping syndrome overview and diagram by MedlinePlus: http://goo.gl/iB6be

Karen is discharged from the hospital after 4 days. She has received information about nutrition, pain control, incisional care, prevention of dumping syndrome, and follow-up appointments. Since Karen is at risk for vitamin and mineral deficiencies, she is started on nutritional supplements. Karen is excited to begin her weight loss journey.

Answers to this chapter begin on page 145.

eResource 4-45: For information regarding postoperative follow-up, consult the Merck Manual [Pathway: www.merckmanuals.com → select "The Merck Manual of Diagnosis and Therapy" → enter "bariatric surgery" into the search field in the upper right corner → select "Follow-up" and review content]

Unfolding Case Study #26 Sarah

Sarah is a 24-year-old female who presents to her primary care provider's (PCP) office with complaints of loss of appetite, nausea, heartburn, and generally not feeling well. She is otherwise healthy with no past medical or surgical history. Her vital signs are temperature 100.2°F, pulse 92, respirations 16, and blood pressure 126/72. The nurse notes that her sclera are slightly yellowed. When the nurse reviews Sarah's past history, she asks if anything has changed. Sarah states that she has been in good health and was recently on a mission trip outside the United States.

Exercise 4-61: *Fill-in*
Considering Sarah's chief complaints and her history of travel outside the United States to a developing country, what is her likely diagnosis? _____

Exercise 4-62: *Fill-in*
The causative organism associated with Sarah's disease process is likely the _____ and the incubation period is _____.

The PCP reviews Sarah's signs and symptoms and completes a physical exam on her. He finds that her liver is slightly enlarged and tender with palpation. He orders some laboratory tests to look at liver function and a specific test to detect hepatitis A virus antibodies. Sarah is also instructed to collect a stool specimen to determine if the hepatitis A antigen is present.

The PCP questions Sarah about what she ate and drank while on her mission trip. Sarah reports that she only drank bottled water, but did eat many local dishes, including some made with shellfish. Sarah is informed that she likely contracted hepatitis A while on her mission trip.

Exercise 4-63: *Fill-in*
Hepatitis A is transmitted primarily through the _____ route by ingesting _____ or _____ contaminated with the virus.

 eResource 4-46: For information regarding hepatitis, consult
■ Merck Manual: [Pathway: www.merckmanuals.com → select "The Merck Manual of Diagnosis and Therapy" → enter "hepatitis" into the search field in the upper right corner → select "Acute Viral Hepatitis" → select "hepatitis A" and review content related to etiology]
■ eMedicinehealth's slideshow, A Visual Guide to Hepatitis: http://goo.gl/B8bCl

Exercise 4-64: *Select all that apply*

Identify other ways in which hepatitis A can be transmitted:

❑ Transfusion of blood products

❑ Infected food handlers

❑ Oral-anal contact during sexual activity

❑ Needle sticks

❑ Poor hygiene

❑ Consuming raw shellfish

Exercise 4-65: *Select all that apply*

Identify other clinical manifestations associated with hepatitis A:

❑ Fatigue

❑ Rashes

❑ Anorexia

❑ Ascites

❑ Dark urine

❑ Aversion to strong odors

eResource 4-47: Within the Merck Manual, review material covering symptoms and signs of hepatitis: [Pathway: www.merckmanuals.com → select "The Merck Manual of Diagnosis and Therapy" → enter "hepatitis" into the search field in the upper right corner → select "Acute Viral Hepatitis" → select "Symptoms and Signs" and review content (both general and virus specific)]

Sarah has her blood drawn at the physician's office and is instructed on how to obtain a stool specimen. She is told to rest as much as possible, with a gradual progression in her activity level.

Sarah is also encouraged to eat a nutritious diet with small, frequent meals recommended. The nurse reviews some important guidelines for managing hepatitis A in the home environment. Sarah is scheduled for a follow-up appointment in 1 week.

Exercise 4-66: *True or false*

Identify whether the following statements about the management of hepatitis A are true or false:

_____ 1. Early studies have shown that a high-protein, high-calorie diet may be beneficial in managing viral hepatitis.

_____ 2. Alcohol should be avoided during the acute illness and for 6 months after recovery.

_____ 3. Good personal hygiene and hand washing are important in preventing the spread of hepatitis to family members.

_____ 4. The hepatitis A vaccine should be given after the acute infection of hepatitis A is past.

Answers to this chapter begin on page 145.

eResource 4-48: Consult Epocrates Online for information regarding patient teaching regarding hepatitis A: [Pathway: https://online.epocrates .com → select "Diseases" → enter "Hepatitis A" in the search field → select "Follow-up" and review content]

Exercise 4-67: *Multiple-choice question*
After educating Sarah about the effects that hepatitis has on the liver, the nurse determines that she understands the information when she states:

    A. "It is okay to use acetaminophen (Tylenol) as much as needed for aches and pains."

    B. "I should talk to my physician before taking any herbal or over-the-counter medications."

    C. "Hepatitis causes very little damage to my liver, so I can start taking more vitamin supplements."

    D. "I will only have one drink on the weekends when I go out with my friends."

At her follow-up appointment, Sarah reports that she is feeling slightly better. Her physician reviews all her laboratory results and confirms that she has hepatitis A. The laboratory results are noted in Table 4-2:

Table 4-2:   Laboratory Results

Laboratory Test	Results
Alanine aminotransferase (ALT)	96 units (High)
Aspartate aminotransferase (AST)	108 units (High)
Serum bilirubin, total	2.9 mg/dL (High)
HAV antibodies	Anti-HAV positive

Exercise 4-68: *Fill-in*
Briefly explain the effect that an elevated bilirubin level has on the body.

_____

_____

_____

 eResource 4-49: To learn more about bilirubin, consult Medscape on your mobile device: [Pathway: Medscape → enter "bilirubin" into the search field → select "bilirubin" and review content]

Answers to this chapter begin on page 145.

Exercise 4-69: *Matching*

Match the type of jaundice in Column A with its cause in Column B.

Column A	Column B
A. Hemolytic jaundice	_____ Extrahepatic obstruction (gallstones)
B. Hepatocellular jaundice	_____ Increased destruction of erythrocytes
C. Obstructive jaundice	_____ Inherited disorder
D. Hereditary hyperbilirubinemia	_____ Damaged liver cells unable to clear bilirubin normally

Exercise 4-70: *Fill-in*

Sarah is likely experiencing _____ jaundice related to liver damage caused by the hepatitis A virus.

e **eResource 4-50:** To review content about jaundice and its management, go to: http://goo.gl/4wzsS

Since many of Sarah's family members travel outside the United States, Sarah asks how they can protect themselves against infection with the hepatitis A virus. The PCP discusses the hepatitis A vaccine with her.

Exercise 4-71: *Select all that apply*

Identify situations/populations where the hepatitis A vaccine may be recommended:

❑ Travel to areas with questionable/poor sanitation

❑ Homosexual men

❑ Dialysis patients

❑ Hemophiliacs

❑ Staff of day care centers

❑ Health care personnel

Exercise 4-72: *Fill-in*

Identify the recommended dosing schedule for the hepatitis A vaccines:

1. Adults _____

2. Children/adolescents 2 to 18 years of age

_____

_____

eResource 4-51: Visit the Society of Teachers of Family Medicine's (STFM) website to download current electronic versions of recommended immunization schedules: [Pathway: www.immunizationed.org → locate the program for your mobile device and download. Note: If you prefer, you can view the pdf versions of the CDC schedules]

Exercise 4-73: *Fill-in*
Briefly explain how people who are exposed to hepatitis A, but have never been vaccinated, are treated.

_____

_____

_____

_____

Sarah is now able to educate her family about hepatitis A prevention. She is progressing toward a full recovery with no anticipated long-term effects from the viral infection.

 eResource 4-52: Visit Epocrates Online to review recommended patient teaching related to prevention: [Pathway: https://online.epocrates. com → select "Diseases" → enter "Hepatitis A" in the search field → select "Treatment" to review content related to primary and secondary prevention]

Unfolding Case Study #27 ▧ Bob

Bob is a 56-year-old male who was found to have an enlarged, firm liver during a routine physical examination for a new job; however, Bob had no problems or signs/symptoms to report. Laboratory tests, liver/spleen scan, and CT scan were ordered to aid in diagnosis.

 eResource 4-53: To view a video of a CT scan of an abdomen, go to http://goo.gl/0MVHi

Bob is now back in his primary care provider's (PCP) office to find out the results of his tests. His test results are noted in Table 4-3:

Table 4-3: Laboratory Results

Laboratory Test	Results
Alanine aminotransferase (ALT)	100 units/L (High)
Aspartate aminotransferase (AST)	105 units/L (High)
Gamma-glutamyltranspeptidase (GGT)	60 units/L (High)
Alkaline phosphatase	200 units/L (High)

Answers to this chapter begin on page 145.

The results of Bob's laboratory tests, liver/spleen scan, and CT scan all support the diagnosis of hepatic cirrhosis. Since he is free of major signs and symptoms, Bob is currently compensating for his disease. He has many questions about what this diagnosis means.

Exercise 4-74: *Matching*
Match the type of cirrhosis in Column A with its cause in Column B.

Column A	Column B
A. Alcoholic cirrhosis	_____ Late result of acute viral hepatitis
B. Postnecrotic cirrhosis	_____ Results from chronic biliary obstruction
C. Biliary cirrhosis	_____ Results from chronic alcoholism

Exercise 4-75: *Fill-in*
The major causative factor of fatty liver and cirrhosis is _____ although _____ also contributes to liver destruction.

Exercise 4-76: *Fill-in*
Briefly explain why cirrhotic livers are described as having a hobnail appearance.

_____

_____

_____

_____

 eResource 4-54: Consult Epocrates Online to review content related to cirrhosis: [Pathway: https://online.epocrates.com → under the "Diseases" tab, enter "cirrhosis" in the search field and review the content and image library]

Bob asks why he is not having problems associated with his disease, and his PCP explains the progression of cirrhosis, including how he is currently compensating. The PCP asks Bob about his alcohol intake. Bob states that he doesn't drink that much, maybe two beers on some days, but his PCP strongly recommends that he stop drinking to slow the progression of his liver disease. Bob is given further instructions, including a follow-up appointment.

 eResource 4-55: Additional patient education material, focusing upon self-care at home, can be found at eMedicinehealth.com: http://goo.gl/Fr6nT

Exercise 4-77: *Select all that apply*

Identify signs and symptoms associated with compensated cirrhosis:

❑ Hypotension

❑ Palmar erythema

❑ Vascular spiders

❑ Vague morning indigestion

❑ Jaundice

❑ Ascites

Bob does not keep his follow-up appointment, nor does he stop using alcohol. Several years pass without him having any health problems until today when he is admitted to the hospital with confusion and restlessness. Bob's wife helps the nurse to complete his admission history. She states that Bob has been healthy except for the doctor saying he had cirrhosis several years ago. The nurse questions if Bob continues to use alcohol; the wife indicates that he drinks about a six-pack of beer a day. On physical assessment, the nurse notes that Bob is very restless; disoriented to person, place, and time; and has a distended abdomen. Laboratory tests are ordered, and the PCP is notified of Bob's arrival to the nursing unit.

Exercise 4-78: *Fill-in*

Identify five functions of the liver:

1. _____

2. _____

3. _____

4. _____

5. _____

e   **eResource 4-56:** To learn more about liver function, view:
    ■ *Liver Health: How Does the Liver Function:* http://youtu.be/RsPzIqcVaoY
    ■ An animation demonstrating the function of the liver: http://youtu.be/ tat0QYxlCbo

The PCP arrives at the unit; he reviews Bob's laboratory results and conducts a physical examination before talking to Bob's wife. All of his liver function tests (ALT, AST, GGT, and alkaline phosphatase) are abnormally elevated. The ammonia level is 210 mcg/dL. The PCP explains to Bob's wife that as a result of his decompensating cirrhosis, he now has ascites and hepatic encephalopathy. As the PCP writes treatment orders, the wife asks the nurse to further explain what is happening with Bob.

Exercise 4-79: *Select all that apply*

Identify clinical manifestations associated with ascites:

❑ Increased abdominal girth

❑ Hematemesis

Answers to this chapter begin on page 145.

❑ Rapid weight gain

❑ Distended veins on abdominal wall

❑ Shortness of breath

❑ Asterixis

eResource 4-57: To help Bob better understand ascites, the primary care provider provides:
- ▣ Patient education materials: http://goo.gl/9927I
- ▣ A video explaining ascites: http://youtu.be/pvuvlcgbG90

Exercise 4-80: *Select all that apply*

Identify clinical manifestations associated with hepatic encephalopathy:

❑ Melena

❑ Change in mood and sleep patterns

❑ Constructional apraxia

❑ Fetor hepaticus

❑ Hypotension

❑ Asterixis

eResource 4-58: For a more detailed overview of hepatic encephalopathy:
- ▣ Watch a video presentation: http://youtu.be/WOcFuVa4VoY
- ▣ Visit Medscape:
  - ▣ Online: [Pathway: www.medscape.org → Under the tab "Reference," select "References & Tools" → enter "hepatic encephalopathy" into the search field and review content]
  - ▣ On your mobile device, you can access the same information: [Pathway: Medscape → enter "hepatic encephalopathy" into the search field and review content]

Exercise 4-81: *True or false*

Identify whether the following statements about ascites and hepatic encephalopathy are true or false:

_____ 1. The presence of fluid in the abdomen (ascites) can be confirmed by assessing for a fluid wave or percussing for shifting dullness.

_____ 2. In stage 4 of hepatic encephalopathy, patients are comatose with markedly abnormal electroencephalograms.

_____ 3. Furosemide (Lasix), an aldosterone-blocking agent, is first-line therapy in the treatment of ascites.

_____ 4. Some restriction of protein is usually needed in patients who are comatose or have encephalopathy.

Answers to this chapter begin on page 145.

The nurse reviews the treatment orders, which include:

- Bed rest
- 2-g sodium diet with protein restriction of 1.0 g/kg/day
- Dietician consult
- Neurological checks every 2 hours
- Daily weights
- Accurate intake/output every shift
- BMP and ammonia levels every a.m.
- Spironolactone (Aldactone) 100 mg PO bid
- Lactulose (Cephulac) 30 mL PO bid

 eResource 4-59: Consult Epocrates Online for detailed information related to these prescribed medications: [Pathway: https://online .epocrates.com → select "drugs" → enter each medication in the search field and review content]

Exercise 4-82: *Multiple-choice question*

When Bob's wife asks why he is on a 2-g sodium, protein-restricted diet, the nurse's best response is:

    A. "That is not important right now; he will not go home on this diet."
    B. "The salt and protein restriction will allow his liver to heal."
    C. "The restrictions reduce fluid retention and ammonia levels, thus improving his symptoms."
    D. "This diet is prescribed to help him lose some weight."

Exercise 4-83: *Select all that apply*

Identify causes of increased ammonia levels in patients with hepatic cirrhosis:

    ❑ Antibiotic administration
    ❑ Gastrointestinal bleeding
    ❑ High-protein diets
    ❑ Hyperkalemia
    ❑ Bacterial infections
    ❑ Acidosis

Exercise 4-84: *Multiple-choice question*

After educating Bob's wife about his protein-restricted diet, the nurse determines that his wife understands the information when she states:

    A. "Protein should be eliminated from the diet to prevent increasing ammonia levels."
    B. "Animal protein is usually better tolerated than vegetable or dairy protein."

Answers to this chapter begin on page 145.

    C. "Larger, less frequent meals are more effective in preventing protein loading."

    D. "Protein intake can be increased if mental status is improving, but should be reduced if neurological signs/symptoms return."

Bob's wife has a clearer understanding of what is happening with her husband. Once Bob recovers, he and his wife will require a lot of teaching to prevent recurrent episodes of encephalopathy. It is of utmost importance that Bob stop his alcohol intake completely to prevent further liver damage.

 eResource 4-60: Consult Epocrates Online for detailed information related to discharge teaching and follow-up for Bob and his wife: [Pathway: https://online.epocrates.com → select "Diseases" → enter "cirrhosis" in the search field → select "Follow-Up" and review content]

Unfolding Case Study #28 ▨ Patrick

Patrick is a 40-year-old male who came to the emergency department (ED) with complaints of nausea and right upper quadrant pain that goes through to his back. The pain woke him up during the night and it has been constant for 4 hours. Patrick reports that he felt fine yesterday, and he and his family went out for Mexican food last evening.

Exercise 4-85: *Fill-in*
Based on Patrick's presenting signs and symptoms, it is likely that he is having a problem with either _____ or _____.

The primary care provider (PCP) orders an ultrasound of the gallbladder, which confirms the presence of stones.

 eResource 4-61: For an overview of the anatomy of the gallbladder and this procedure, view the following:
▨ Gallbladder Ultrasound Part 1: http://youtu.be/FY3dBuQV03w
▨ Gallbladder Ultrasound Part 2: http://youtu.be/L3e-YdQRa-A

Exercise 4-86: *Fill-in*
Briefly explain how the gallbladder functions and delivers bile to the duodenum.

_____

_____

_____

Exercise 4-87: *Fill-in*
Briefly explain the difference between cholecystitis and cholelithiasis.

_____

_____

_____

Answers to this chapter begin on page 145.

Patrick is diagnosed with cholelithiasis and a surgeon is consulted. He remains extremely restless and reports his pain level as 8 out of 10. The PCP orders an IV line started and hydromorphone (Dilaudid) 1.5 mg IV every 3 hours PRN.

 eResource 4-62: To learn more about drug and associated precautions, consult Skyscape's RxDrugs on your mobile device: [Pathway: Skyscape → select "RxDrugs" → enter "dilaudid" into the search field → select "injectable" and review content]

Exercise 4-88: *Select all that apply*
Identify common risk factors for cholelithiasis:
- ❑ Obesity
- ❑ Male gender
- ❑ High-fat diets
- ❑ Rapid weight loss
- ❑ Diabetes mellitus
- ❑ Age less than 40

Exercise 4-89: *Select all that apply*
Identify clinical manifestations associated with cholelithiasis:
- ❑ Biliary colic
- ❑ Jaundice
- ❑ Change in urine and stool color
- ❑ Melena
- ❑ Diarrhea
- ❑ Pruritus

 eResource 4-63: To learn more about clinical manifestations of cholelithiasis, go to Medscape:
- ▣ Online: [Pathway: www.medscape.org → Under the tab "Reference," select "References & Tools" → enter "cholelithiasis" into the search field and review content]
- ▣ On a mobile device: [Pathway: Medscape → enter "cholelithiasis" into the search field and review content. Note: Be sure to review images]

Exercise 4-90: *Calculation*
Order: hydromorphone (Dilaudid) 1.5 mg IV every 3 hours PRN
    Dilaudid is supplied as 2 mg in 1 mL.
Calculate the dose of Dilaudid to be given in mL: _____

 eResource 4-64: Use MedCalc's Online Calculator to verify your understanding: [Pathway: www.medcalc.com → select "Fluids/Electrolytes" → select "IV Rate" and enter information into fields]

Answers to this chapter begin on page 145.

Patrick is seen by the general surgeon and informed that he will need surgery to remove his gallbladder and the obstructing stone that is causing his symptoms. Patrick will be admitted to the surgical unit, and surgery will be performed the following day. The surgeon is planning on performing a laparoscopic cholecystectomy. Patrick is being kept NPO. IV fluids are ordered: 0.9% NaCl at 100 mL/hr.

Exercise 4-91: *True or false*

Identify whether the following statements about the medical management of cholelithiasis are true or false:

_____ 1. Nonsurgical treatments provide only a temporary solution and are associated with persistent symptoms and recurrent stone formation.

_____ 2. Ursodeoxycholic acid is effective in dissolving or reducing the size of pigment stones.

_____ 3. Extracorporeal shock wave lithotripsy, which uses shock waves to break up stones, is the treatment of choice for gallbladder disease.

_____ 4. Laparoscopic cholecystectomies have decreased the surgical risks, length of hospital stay, and recovery period compared to the open cholecystectomies.

e **eResource 4-65:** For better understanding of this surgical procedure, review the following:
- Laparoscopic cholecystectomy: http://goo.gl/JBFXh
- On your mobile device, open Medscape [Pathway: Medscape → enter "cholecystectomy" into the search field and review content. Be sure to view the media library]

Exercise 4-92: *Select all that apply*

Identify foods that should be avoided in patients who have intolerances to fatty foods and vague gastrointestinal symptoms associated with biliary disease:

❑ Skim milk
❑ Mashed potatoes
❑ Fried foods
❑ Cheese
❑ Bread
❑ Alcohol

On the following day, Patrick has his laparoscopic cholecystectomy. Postoperatively, his vital signs are stable and his pain is under control. Discharge is planned for early the next morning.

Answers to this chapter begin on page 145.

Exercise 4-93: *Fill-in*

Identify three potential nursing diagnoses for the patient postoperatively following gallbladder surgery:

1. _____

2. _____

3. _____

Exercise 4-94: *Multiple-choice question*

When Patrick's wife asks why he is having pain in his right shoulder, the nurse's best response is:

    A. "The pain is related to how he was positioned during surgery."

    B. "This pain may indicate that he still has a stone lodged somewhere."

    C. "This pain is referred from the site where his gallbladder was removed."

    D. "Pain occurs in this location from the gas used to inflate the abdomen during surgery."

Patrick is encouraged to begin ambulating, and sequential compression devices are ordered for when he is in bed. The nurse encourages incentive spirometry 10 breaths every 1 to 2 hours. Patrick is started on a full liquid diet and may advance to a soft diet as tolerated.

 eResource 4-66: To reinforce her teaching, the nurse shows Patrick a video demonstrating the proper technique for using an incentive spirometry, view http://youtu.be/VHN5zPaw96w

The following day, Patrick is discharged home.

Exercise 4-95: *Fill-in*

Briefly explain why patients are placed on a low-fat diet following surgery.

_____

_____

_____

Exercise 4-96: *Multiple-choice question*

After educating Patrick about his activity restrictions after discharge, the nurse determines that he understands the information when he states:

    A. "I should do nothing but rest the next couple of weeks."

    B. "I should avoid showering the next 3 days."

    C. "I need to wait 3 to 4 days before driving."

    D. "I can't wait to pick up and hug my 4-year-old when I get home."

Answers to this chapter begin on page 145.

Exercise 4-97: *Multiple-choice question*

As Patrick asks further questions about wound care, the nurse determines that he needs further instruction when he states:

    A. "I need to call the physician if I have a fever or notice redness or drainage at the site."

    B. "I should change these Steri-Strips daily and apply new dressings."

    C. "These wounds can be washed with soap and water."

    D. "I can leave these wounds open to air."

After returning home, Patrick recovered from his surgery without complications. He returned to his job after 2 weeks.

Unfolding Case Study #29   Roy

Roy is a 56-year-old male who presents to the emergency department (ED) with severe midepigastric abdominal pain, nausea, and vomiting. He has a history of hypertension. On physical assessment, he is noted to have abdominal distension and tenderness with palpation. The physician questions Roy about his social history with alcohol, smoking, and illicit drugs. He admits to drinking a few beers and smoking a pack of cigarettes every day. The physician orders laboratory tests and a CT scan of the abdomen. Roy's wife privately speaks to the physician to inform him that Roy actually drinks at least a six-pack of beer daily with an even higher intake on the weekends. This past weekend, Roy and his friends drank heavily while watching football.

Exercise 4-98: *Fill-in*

Based on Roy's presenting signs and symptoms and his significant alcohol history, it is possible that Roy has _____.

Exercise 4-99: *Fill-in*

Identify three digestive enzymes secreted by the exocrine pancreas and their function:

    1. _____

    2. _____

    3. _____

Exercise 4-100: *Select all that apply*

Identify clinical manifestations associated with acute pancreatitis:

    ❑ Acute, severe abdominal pain that occurs 24 to 48 hours after a heavy meal or alcohol intake

    ❑ Hypercalcemia

    ❑ Nausea unrelieved by vomiting

    ❑ Hypervolemia

Answers to this chapter begin on page 145.

❑ Ecchymosis in the flank or umbilical area

❑ Abdominal guarding

 eResource 4-67: To learn more about the clinical presentation of acute pancreatitis, consult the Merck Manual: [Pathway: www.merckmanuals. com → select "The Merck Manual of Diagnosis and Therapy" → enter "acute pancreatitis" into the search field in the upper right corner → select "Overview of GI Bleeding" → select "Interpretation of findings"]

Roy's laboratory test results are back and the abnormal results are noted in Table 4-4:

Table 4-4:   Laboratory Results

Laboratory Test	Results
Amylase	300 units/L (High)
Lipase	210 units/L (High)
White blood cells (WBCs)	16,000/mm³ (High)
Glucose	168 mg/dL (High)
Calcium	8.1 mg/dL (Low)

The physician explains to Roy and his wife that Roy has acute pancreatitis and will need to be admitted to a medical floor for treatment.

Exercise 4-101: *Fill-in*

Identify why the above laboratory tests are abnormal in relation to the diagnosis of acute pancreatitis:

1. Amylase:_____

2. Lipase:_____

3. White blood cells:_____

4. Glucose:_____

5. Calcium:_____

 eResource 4-68: Consult Stedman's Laboratory Reference Range Values: http://goo.gl/tXI3a

Exercise 4-102: *Multiple-choice question*

When Roy's wife asks how acute pancreatitis develops, the nurse's best response is:

A. "Acute pancreatitis is autodigestion of the pancreas by its own enzymes; it occurs most often with gallstones or long-term alcohol use."

B. "Acute pancreatitis is most often caused by tumors of the pancreas or intestines."

C. "Acute pancreatitis occurs when the pancreas is damaged by frequently eating spicy, hot foods combined with alcohol."

D. "Acute pancreatitis occurs in patients with hypertension who have blood pressures that are high for prolonged periods."

Answers to this chapter begin on page 145.

eResource 4-69: For an overview of pancreatitis, view *What Is Pancreatitis?* http://youtu.be/iA7cwCexs6w

Roy is admitted to a medical unit with the following orders:

- Bed rest
- Incentive spirometer 10 breaths every 1 to 2 hours
- NPO (strict)
- IV fluids of Lactated Ringer's at 125 mL/hr
- Ondansetron (Zofran) 2 mg IV every 6 hours PRN
- Morphine 2 mg IV every 2 hours PRN
- Fingerstick blood sugars every 6 hours
- Sliding-scale insulin coverage with lispro (Humalog)

Exercise 4-103: *Fill-in*
Briefly explain why strict NPO is enforced for patients with pancreatitis.

_____

_____

_____

Exercise 4-104: *Calculation*
Order: Morphine 2 mg IV every 2 hours PRN
     Morphine is supplied as 5 mg in 2 mL.
Calculate the dose of morphine to be given in mL: _____

 eResource 4-70: Use MedCalc to verify your answer: [Pathway: www .medcalc.com → select "Fluids/Electrolytes" → select "IV Rate" and enter information into fields]

Exercise 4-105: *Calculation*
Order: Sliding-scale insulin coverage with lispro (Humalog)
     Formula: For blood sugars greater than 150 mg/dL: (Blood sugar − 100) divided by 30.
     Fingerstick blood sugar is 194.
Calculate the amount of Humalog to be given in units: _____

 eResource 4-71: For additional information regarding sliding-scale therapy, review http://goo.gl/CPldH

Exercise 4-106: *True or false*
Identify whether the following statements about the medical management of acute pancreatitis are true or false:

     _____ 1. Patients with acute pancreatitis require aggressive respiratory care because of the high risk of pulmonary infiltrates, effusions, and atelectasis.

Answers to this chapter begin on page 145.

———— 2. Nasogastric tubes are routinely ordered in patients with acute pancreatitis in order to remove gastric secretions.

———— 3. Hypotension and decreased urine output are treated with fluids and blood products to replace fluid lost.

———— 4. After recovery from acute pancreatitis, patients are advised to avoid high-fat foods, heavy meals, and alcohol.

Roy requires frequent medication for pain and nausea. Roy's wife is very concerned and remains at his bedside. She frequently asks questions to learn more about acute pancreatitis and its treatment. The physician decides to start Roy on morphine patient-controlled analgesia (PCA).

Exercise 4-107: *Multiple-choice question*
After educating Roy and his wife about the need to turn and reposition every 2 hours, the nurse determines that the wife understands the information when she states:

A. "Turning every 2 hours will help to reduce the pain he is feeling."

B. "Getting out of bed and walking is actually the best for him."

C. "Frequent position changes help prevent skin breakdown and lung problems."

D. "Keeping him flat in bed will help him to breathe better."

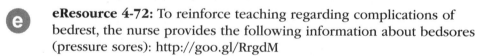 **eResource 4-72:** To reinforce teaching regarding complications of bedrest, the nurse provides the following information about bedsores (pressure sores): http://goo.gl/RrgdM

Exercise 4-108: *Multiple-choice question*
When Roy's wife asks how PCA works, the nurse's best response is:

A. "The patient or family can push the button at any time to deliver pain medication."

B. "PCA pumps allow patients to control administration of their medication, often resulting in better pain relief."

C. "PCA pumps improve pain control, but increase the risk of overdose."

D. "The family needs to ensure the patient is breathing well before the button is pushed."

eResource 4-73: To reinforce patient teaching regarding morphine, consult Medscape on your mobile device: [Pathway: Medscape → enter "Morphine" into the search field and review content]

Answers

Exercise 4-1: *Fill-in*

The nurse is aware that Craig's signs and symptoms are consistent with the clinical manifestations associated with: <u>**peptic ulcer disease**</u>.

Exercise 4-2: *Select all that apply*

Identify factors that can cause and/or contribute to gastrointestinal ulceration:

☒ ***H. pylori* —YES, this gram-negative bacteria can cause peptic ulcers.**

☒ **Caffeinated beverages—YES, this may increase HCl secretion in the stomach, which may contribute to ulcer formation.**

☒ **Milk ingestion—YES, this may increase HCl secretion in the stomach, which may contribute to ulcer formation.**

❏ High protein diets—NO, although spicy foods may worsen ulcers.

☒ **Excessive smoking—YES, this may increase HCl secretion in the stomach, which may contribute to ulcer formation.**

Exercise 4-3: *Fill-in*

Identify Craig's risk factors for peptic ulcer disease and the rationale for how they place him at risk:

1. <u>**Age (40)—ulcers occur most frequently between 40 to 60 years of age.**</u>
2. <u>**High stress job—may cause excessive secretion of HCl in the stomach.**</u>
3. <u>**Alcohol use—may increase secretion of HCl with chronic use (may not apply to Craig).**</u>
4. <u>**Ibuprofen use—inhibits secretion of mucus that protects the gastroduodenal mucosa; occurs more with chronic use (may not apply to Craig).**</u>

Exercise 4-4: *Select all that apply*

Identify clinical manifestations associated with peptic ulcer disease:

❏ Diffuse abdominal tenderness—NO, pain/tenderness is usually localized to the epigastrium.

☒ **Pyrosis—YES, this is a burning sensation that moves from the stomach to the mouth.**

☒ **Melena—YES, this is tarry stool that indicates upper gastrointestinal bleeding.**

❏ Frequent vomiting—NO, this is not common unless there is a pyloric obstruction.

☒ **Sour eructation—YES**

Exercise 4-5: *Matching*

Match the type of ulcer in Column A with its common characteristics in Column B. Answers in Column A can be used more than once.

Column A	Column B
A. Duodenal ulcer	__A__ 80% of ulcers are this type
B. Gastric ulcer	__B__ Usually occurs in people older than 50 years
	__A__ Associated with hypersecretion of HCl
	__A__ Pain occurs 2 to 3 hours after meal
	__B__ Ingestion of food does not help pain
	__B__ Hematemesis more common

Exercise 4-6: *True or false*

Identify whether the following statements about Hemoccult II stool testing for occult blood are true or false:

__True__ 1. Aspirin and nonsteroidal anti-inflammatory drugs (NSAIDs) may cause a false-positive result.

__True__ 2. Turnips and horseradish should be avoided for 72 hours prior to testing because they may cause a false-positive result.

__False__ 3. Vitamin C supplements may cause a false-positive result.

__True__ 4. Red meat may cause a false-positive result if ingested within 72 hours prior to testing.

Exercise 4-7: *Fill-in*

Identify three nursing diagnoses for the patient with peptic ulcer disease:

1. **Acute pain related to gastric acid exposure on damaged mucosa**
2. **Imbalanced nutrition related to changes in diet**
3. **Anxiety related to unknown and acute illness**
4. **Knowledge deficit related to management of disease process**

Exercise 4-8: *Multiple-choice question*

After educating Craig on the endoscopy procedure and pre-procedure instructions, the nurse determines that he understands the information when he states:

A. "I will have to stay in the hospital overnight after this procedure."—NO, this can usually be done on an outpatient basis.

B. "I will have to have anesthesia in the operating room during the procedure."—NO, this procedure is usually done in the endoscopy lab with conscious sedation.

C. **"I will be sedated so they can pass a scope down into my stomach and intestine."—YES**

D. "I will have to have my bowels cleaned out prior to this procedure."—NO, an endoscopy only requires that the patient is NPO for 8 hours prior to the exam.

Exercise 4-9: *Multiple-choice question*

As Craig asks further questions about the endoscopy, the nurse determines that he needs further instruction when he states:

A. **"Since this procedure only takes about 30 minutes, I will be able to drive myself home afterward."—YES, since conscious sedation is given during the procedure, a relative or friend must be available to drive the patient home and preferably stay with him until the following morning.**

B. "I will be sure not to eat or drink anything after midnight tonight."—NO, the patient needs to be NPO for 8 hours prior to the exam.

C. "They will spray the back of my throat so I don't gag on the tube."—NO

D. "The doctor will be able to see if I have an ulcer and treat any bleeding."—NO

Exercise 4-10: *Matching*

Match the medication used to treat peptic ulcer disease and *H. pylori* infection in Column A with its action in Column B.

Column A	Column B
A. amoxicillin (Amoxil)	**D** Decreases gastric acid secretion by slowing H^+, K^+-ATPase pump
B. metronidazole (Flagyl)	**A** Bactericidal antibiotic that eradicates *H. pylori*
C. bismuth subsalicylate (Pepto-Bismol)	**B** Synthetic antibacterial and antiprotozoal agent that eradicates *H. pylori*
D. omeprazole (Prilosec)	**C** Suppresses *H. pylori* and assists with healing of mucosal ulcers

Exercise 4-11: *Select all that apply*

Identify recommended dietary changes for patients with peptic ulcer disease:

☐ Replace coffee with decaffeinated coffee—NO, decaffeinated beverages also stimulate acid secretion.

☒ **Avoid extreme temperatures in food and drinks—YES, temperature extremes can stimulate acid secretion.**

☒ **Eat three regular meals per day—YES, this neutralizes acid.**

☐ Increase milk intake—NO, this can stimulate increased acid secretion.

☒ **Avoid alcohol—YES, this can stimulate acid secretion.**

Exercise 4-12: *Multiple-choice question*

Appendicitis is the most common cause of an acute abdomen requiring surgery in the United States related to the fact that the appendix:

A. **is prone to obstruction leading to inflammation, edema, and infection.—YES, the appendix regularly fills with food and empties into the cecum, but it does so inefficiently, leading to obstruction.**

B. has no useful function in the body.—NO

C. is easily inflamed by eating hot, spicy foods.—NO

D. is easily traumatized during contact sports and vehicular accidents.—NO

Exercise 4-13: *Select all that apply*

Identify clinical manifestations exhibited by patients with acute appendicitis:

☒ **Abdominal pain—YES, may begin as a vague epigastric or periumbilical pain, then progresses to a localized right lower quadrant pain.**

☒ **Low-grade fever—YES**

❑ Diarrhea—NO, more likely to have constipation.

❑ Bloody stools—NO

☒ **Nausea with/without vomiting—YES**

☒ **Rovsing's sign—YES, this is when palpation of the left lower quadrant paradoxically causes pain in the right lower quadrant.**

☒ **Rebound tenderness—YES, this is when pain occurs or worsens when pressure is released.**

Exercise 4-14: *Fill-in*

Briefly explain/describe the abdominal pain associated with appendicitis, including whether it is diffuse or localized.

Appendicitis begins as a poorly localized, dull pain in the epigastric or perium-bilical areas. It progresses to become a sharp pain that is localized to the right lower quadrant. If the appendix ruptures, the pain can become more diffuse again.

Exercise 4-15: *Hot spot*

Mark the area where you would elicit pain at McBurney's point in patients with appendicitis:

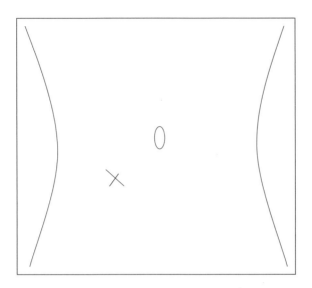

Exercise 4-16: *Fill-in*

Identify the tonicity of the following IV solutions:

1. 0.9% NaCl		**Isotonic**
2. D5NS		**Hypertonic**
3. 0.45% NaCl		**Hypotonic**
4. Lactated Ringer's		**Isotonic**
5. 3% NaCl		**Hypertonic**
6. D5 0.45% NaCl		**Hypertonic**

Exercise 4-17: *Fill-in*

Briefly explain the role of the physician and the nurse in obtaining informed consent.
The physician must provide a clear, simple explanation of the surgery or procedure to be done, including benefits, alternatives, possible risks, complications, and what to expect postoperatively. The nurse clarifies the information, notifies the physician if the patient requires additional information, and witnesses the patient signing the consent form.

Exercise 4-18: *Calculation*

Order: Morphine 4 mg IV every 2 hours PRN for severe pain.

If the morphine is supplied 10 mg per 2 mL, calculate how much morphine you would administer in mL: **0.8 mL**

Exercise 4-19: *Fill-in*
Identify three potential complications that can occur postoperatively in the patient with appendicitis:
1. **Peritonitis**
2. **Pelvic abscess**
3. **Ileus**

Exercise 4-20: *Fill-in*
Identify three nursing diagnoses for the patient with appendicitis:
1. **Acute pain related to inflamed appendix and/or surgical incision.**
2. **Risk for ineffective airway clearance related to depressed respiratory function and pain.**
3. **Risk for infection related to inflamed appendix and/or surgical incision.**
4. **Knowledge deficit related to disease process and postoperative care.**

Exercise 4-21: *Matching*
Match the nursing intervention in Column A with its intended effect/purpose in Column B.

Column A		Column B
A. Diaphragmatic breathing	__E__	Minimizes the risk of postoperative wound infection
B. Leg exercises	__C__	Maintains a comfort level that allows the patient to participate in care
C. Pain control	__A__	Promotes optimal lung expansion and blood oxygenation
D. Splint the incision	__B__	Improves circulation and prevents venous stasis
E. Good hand washing	__D__	Minimizes pressure and pain when coughing

Exercise 4-22: *True or false*
Identify whether the following statements about postoperative nursing interventions are true or false:
__True__ 1. Incentive spirometry is a device that measures and provides feedback on the effectiveness of the patient's breathing.
__False__ 2. Sequential compression devices are effective in maintaining the patient's muscle strength while bedridden.
__True__ 3. Wound assessment and dressing changes are important for early identification of wound infection.

Exercise 4-23: *Multiple-choice question*

After educating Chad on his discharge instructions, the nurse determines that he understands the information when he states:

A. "I should call the physician if I feel nauseated."—NO, only call if nausea is prolonged and affecting food and fluid intake.

B. "I should double my preoperative caloric intake while I am still healing."—NO

C. "I need to avoid heavy lifting until directed by my physician."—YES, this is usually for 2 to 4 weeks postoperative.

D. "I should take a bath daily to soak my abdominal incision."—NO, this increases the risk of contamination and infection with bath water.

Exercise 4-24: *Fill-in*

Identify which of Stephanie's laboratory values are abnormal and whether it is high or low:

1. **Sodium—High**
2. **Chloride—High**
3. **BUN—High**
4. **Creatinine—High**
5. **Osmolality—High**
6. **WBCs—High**

Exercise 4-25: *Fill-in*

Provide a brief explanation of why the blood results may be abnormal.

The fact that the sodium, chloride, BUN, creatinine, and osmolality are all high suggests that the patient is dehydrated. This is supported by the fact that Stephanie has been recently vomiting. The elevated WBCs indicate that there is an infectious process involved.

Exercise 4-26: *Fill-in*

Identify the two types of intestinal obstructions with a brief description and example of both:

1. **Mechanical—an intraluminal obstruction. Examples are adhesions, tumors, or hernias**
2. **Functional—the intestinal musculature cannot propel the contents. Examples are muscular dystrophy, diabetes mellitus, or after bowel manipulation in surgery**

Exercise 4-27: *Matching*

Match the cause of intestinal obstruction in Column A with its description in Column B.

Column A	Column B
A. Adhesions	**C** Bowel twists and turns on itself
B. Intussusception	**D** Bowel protrudes through a weakened abdominal muscle or wall
C. Volvulus	**B** One part of the bowel slips into another part
D. Hernia	**E** A tumor within the intestinal wall protrudes into the lumen
E. Tumor	**A** Bowel becomes adherent to scarred areas after abdominal surgery

Exercise 4-28: *Fill-in*

Identify Stephanie's risk factors for developing an intestinal obstruction with an explanation for why these put her at risk:

The fact that Stephanie has had three surgical procedures (cholecystectomy, two cesarean births) puts her at risk for adhesions, which can in turn, cause intestinal obstruction.

Exercise 4-29: *Select all that apply*

Identify clinical manifestations exhibited by patients with small bowel obstructions:

☒ **Crampy, wave-like abdominal pain—YES, this is often the initial symptom.**

❑ Increased flatus—NO, flatus will be absent.

☒ **Fecal vomiting—YES, if the obstruction is complete, peristalsis can reverse direction.**

☒ **Abdominal distension—YES, it is worse the lower the obstruction in the gastrointestinal tract.**

☒ **Dehydration—YES, fluid absorption decreases with the obstruction.**

❑ Large, hardened bowel movements—NO, there is no passage of stool.

Exercise 4-30: *Ordering*

Number in order the steps required for insertion of a nasogastric tube:

4 Explain the purpose of the tube and procedure for insertion.

8 Lubricate the tube with water-soluble lubricant.

1 Confirm the physician's order.

6 Sit the patient upright in bed.

9 Instruct the patient to lower head as tube reaches nasopharynx.

2 Gather supplies.

11 Confirm tube placement.

3 Identify the patient.

__10__ Instruct the patient to swallow as tube is advanced.

__12__ Secure tube to nose.

__7__ Measure from the tip of the nose to the earlobe to the xiphoid process.

__5__ Apply clean gloves.

Exercise 4-31: *True or false*

Identify whether the following statements about assessing nasogastric tube placement are true or false:

__True__ 1. X-ray visualization of the tube tip is the most accurate method for verifying placement.

__False__ 2. Air auscultation is a traditional method that has been shown to be a reliable indicator of tube placement.

__False__ 3. Visual assessment of aspirate color is effective in ruling out respiratory placement.

__True__ 4. Gastric pH measurements are affected by continuous tube feedings and proton pump inhibitors.

Exercise 4-32: *Multiple-choice question*

Decompression of the bowel is successful in most cases, but surgery may be warranted if:

A. The patient has had an NG tube for 12 hours.—NO

B. The NG tube is draining bile-colored contents.—NO

C. The patient is uncomfortable with the NG tube.—NO

D. The bowel is completely obstructed and causing necrosis.—YES, this increases the risk of rupture or perforation, resulting in peritonitis.

Exercise 4-33: *Fill-in*

Briefly explain/describe a clear liquid diet, including indications for use with Stephanie: **A clear liquid diet includes any transparent liquid that can be poured at room temperature. It provides fluid and energy. This diet requires minimal digestive action, so it is prescribed as a first step in reintroducing oral intake following surgery and/or gastrointestinal problems. This diet is inadequate in necessary nutrients and should only be used short term.**

Exercise 4-34: *Select all that apply*

Identify foods/liquids permitted with a clear liquid diet:

☒ **Ginger ale—YES, clear carbonated beverages are permitted.**

☒ **Popsicles—YES**

☐ Orange juice—NO, this is not transparent.

☐ Milk—NO, this is not transparent.

☒ **Clear broth—YES**

Exercise 4-35: *Fill-in*
Identify John's risk factors for colorectal cancer:

1. **Age**

2. **Obesity**

3. **History of polyps**

4. **History of smoking**

5. **Family history of colon cancer**

Exercise 4-36: *Select all that apply*
Identify additional risk factors for colorectal cancer:

☐ Benign prostatic hyperplasia—NO

☒ **High-fat, high-protein, low-fiber diet—YES**

☐ Hypertension—NO

☒ **History of heavy alcohol use—YES**

☒ **History of inflammatory bowel disease—YES**

Exercise 4-37: *Fill-in*
The most common presenting symptom of colorectal cancer is **a change in bowel habits** and the second most common is **blood in or on the stools.**

Exercise 4-38: *Matching*
Match the location of the lesion or tumor in Column A with its commonly associated symptoms in Column B. Answers in Column A can be used more than once.

Column A	Column B
A. Right-sided lesions	__B__ Cramping pain
B. Left-sided lesions	__C__ Ineffective, painful straining at stool
C. Rectal lesions	__A__ Melena
	__B__ Abdominal distension
	__B__ Narrow stools
	__C__ Feeling of incomplete evacuation after bowel movement

Exercise 4-39: *Multiple-choice question*
Lavage solutions, such as GoLYTELY, are effective in cleansing the bowel for optimal visualization, but side effects include:
A. Nausea, vomiting, and fluid overload—NO, fluid deficit/loss is more likely.
B. Bloating, constipation, and painful straining at stools—NO, the effect of GoLYTELY is to cleanse the bowel of stool.

C. Nausea, cramps, and constipation—NO, the effect of GoLYTELY is to cleanse the bowel of stool.

D. **Cramps, abdominal fullness, and fluid/electrolyte imbalances—YES, fluid/ electrolyte imbalances can occur if adequate fluid, electrolyte, and caloric intake is not maintained during the prep.**

Exercise 4-40: *Fill-in*

Briefly explain how carcinoembryonic antigen (CEA) is used as a prognostic predictor of cancer and the effectiveness of treatment:

CEA is a protein not normally found in healthy people, so when detected, it indicates that cancer is present. With effective treatment, CEA levels will decrease and even return to normal with complete excision of tumors. A later increase in CEA suggests that cancer has returned.

Exercise 4-41: *Select all that apply*

Identify interventions used to monitor patients after colonoscopy to ensure a safe recovery:

☒ **Monitor oxygen saturation—YES, respiratory depression can occur related to medications administered during the procedure.**

☐ Check vital signs hourly × 4, then every 4 hours—NO, vitals sign are usually checked every 15 minutes × 4, every 30 minutes × 4, and then every 1 hour × 4.

☒ **Monitor for worsening abdominal pain or distension—YES, this could indicate bowel perforation.**

☒ **Monitor level of consciousness—YES, after the procedure, the patient should start to become increasingly awake and alert as the medication wears off.**

Exercise 4-42: *Multiple-choice question*

When John states that he is scared that he is going to die, the nurse's best response is:

A. "Don't worry; everything is going to be okay."—NO, this is false reassurance.

B. "I know someone who had cancer; I can tell you their story."—NO

C. **"It must be very frightening for you to have just received this diagnosis."— YES, this acknowledges the patient's feelings and leaves an opening for him to continue.**

D. "I can try to find someone to talk with you further."—NO, this sends the message that you don't have time or are uncomfortable, and the patient will likely leave at that point.

Exercise 4-43: *Fill-in*

John is put on a diet high in calories, protein, and carbohydrates and low in residue after his appointment. Twenty-four hours before surgery, he is changed to a full liquid diet. Briefly explain the rationale behind these dietary orders:

John is initially put on a diet high in calories, protein, and carbohydrates to optimize his nutritional status prior to surgery. The low residue diet minimizes any cramping by decreasing excessive peristalsis. A full liquid diet is prescribed for 24 to 48 hours before surgery to decrease stool bulk and facilitate bowel cleansing.

Exercise 4-44: *Multiple-choice question*

When John asks why he needs to take an antibiotic the day before surgery, the nurse's best response is:

A. "This is done prophylactically to prevent infection."—NO, this is terminology the patient probably won't understand and it doesn't always prevent infection.

B. **"The cephalexin (Keflex) will reduce the bacteria in your intestines before surgery."—YES, this is understandable and then it can be further explained that this reduces the risk of infection.**

C. "The tumor is already causing an infection in your body."—NO

D. "It is given the day before surgery to start your antibiotics early."—NO

Exercise 4-45: *Matching*

Match the colostomy site in Column A with its expected fecal output in Column B.

Column A	Column B	
A. Ascending colostomy	**B**	Unformed stool
B. Transverse colostomy	**D**	Formed stool
C. Descending colostomy	**A**	Fluid stool
D. Sigmoid colostomy	**C**	Semi-formed stool

Exercise 4-46: *Select all that apply*

Identify foods that cause excessive gas and odor and should therefore be avoided:

☒ **Asparagus—YES**

❑ Milk—NO

☒ **Eggs—YES**

☒ **Beans—YES**

❑ Tomatoes—NO

☒ **Cabbage—YES**

Exercise 4-47: *True or false*

Identify whether the following statements about colostomy care are true or false:

__True__ 1. A stoma that is beefy red or pink in color is healthy and indicates good circulation.

__False__ 2. The colostomy should begin functioning with 12 hours of surgery.

__False__ 3. Colostomy appliances should be changed every 24 hours to avoid leakage.

__True__ 4. Empty the colostomy appliance when it is one-third full to prevent the appliance from separating from the skin.

Exercise 4-48: *Calculation*

Calculate Karen's body mass index (BMI) using the following formula:

$$BMI = 703 \times weight\ in\ pounds/(height\ in\ inches)^2$$
__49.1__

Exercise 4-49: *Calculation*

Calculate Karen's ideal body weight using the following formula:

❏ Allow 100 pounds for 5 feet of height

❏ Add 5 pounds for each additional inch over 5 feet

❏ Subtract 10% for small frames; add 10% for large frames

125 pounds +/− 12.5 pounds

Exercise 4-50: *Select all that apply*

Identify health risks associated with morbid obesity:

❏ Chronic obstructive pulmonary disease (COPD)—NO

☒ **Diabetes—YES**

☒ **Heart disease—YES**

☒ **Gallbladder disease—YES**

❏ Urinary tract infections—NO

☒ **Sleep apnea—YES**

Exercise 4-51: *True or false*

Identify whether the following statements about lifestyle and food intake are true or false:

__False__ 1. People who regularly skip breakfast are less likely to be obese.

__False__ 2. Eating meals out is associated with a lower food intake.

__True__ 3. The faster food is eaten, the greater the food intake.

__True__ 4. The greater the variety of food, the more kilocalories consumed.

Exercise 4-52: *Fill-in*

A weight loss diet should be reduced in total kilocalories, but also meet the following requirements:

1. Carbohydrates __45__ % of kilocalories
2. Fat __20__ % of kilocalories
3. Protein __10__ % of kilocalories
4. __25__ % of kilocalories open to negotiation
5. Fiber __24–35__ grams

Exercise 4-53: *Multiple-choice question*

After discussing exercise for weight loss, the primary care provider (PCP) determines that Karen needs further instruction when she states:

A. "I should begin with 30 to 45 minutes of exercise 3 to 5 days per week."—NO, this moderate level of activity is recommended.

B. "I need to drink water before, during, and after exercise, especially in hot weather."—NO, this is recommended in order to prevent dehydration.

C. "In order to maintain weight loss, I will have to continue exercising even after reaching my goal."—NO, this is correct.

D. "The only way to continue to lose weight is by running."—YES, there are other effective forms of exercise, like swimming.

Exercise 4-54: *Fill-in*

Identify five behavior modification techniques recommended to facilitate weight loss:

1. **Keep a food diary of all food intake.**
2. **Keep a weekly graph of weight loss/gain.**
3. **Sit down at a table while eating.**
4. **Decide beforehand what you will eat at a restaurant.**
5. **Drink a glass of water before each meal.**
6. **Try to be the last one finished eating.**
7. **Make an agreement with yourself for a meaningful reward.**
8. **Do not reward yourself with food.**
9. **Imagine yourself ordering a healthy choice at a fast food restaurant.**
10. **View exercise as a means of controlling hunger.**

Exercise 4-55: *Fill-in*

Two potential side effects associated with the new weight loss medication Qsymia are **heart palpitations** and **birth defects.**

Exercise 4-56: *Fill-in*

Bariatric surgeries aid in weight loss through **restricting the ability to eat (restrictive procedure), interfering with nutrient absorption (malabsorptive procedure),** or both.

Exercise 4-57: *True or false*

Identify whether the following statements about selection criteria for bariatric surgery are true or false:

__False__ 1. To be eligible for bariatric surgery, all patients must have a BMI greater than 40 kg/m².

__True__ 2. Patients are expected to adhere to postoperative care, medical management, and follow-up visits after bariatric surgery.

__True__ 3. A patient will be excluded from surgery if he or she is unable to comprehend the risks, benefits, and lifestyle changes required.

__False__ 4. Patients are not required to have a history of failed dieting or other nonsurgical attempts at weight loss prior to surgical intervention.

Exercise 4-58: *Select all that apply*

Identify common complications that can occur after bariatric surgery:

☒ **Bleeding—YES**

☒ **Leaking from anastomosis site—YES, this can lead to infection.**

❑ Unstable blood sugars—NO

❑ Dehydration—NO

☒ **Nausea—YES, often results from overfilling the stomach pouch.**

☒ **Change in bowel function—YES, diarrhea or constipation may occur.**

Exercise 4-59: *Select all that apply*

Identify dietary guidelines for the patient post bariatric surgery:

☒ **Eat 3 to 6 small meals per day—YES, approximately 600–800 calories per day.**

❑ Choose foods low in calories and nutrients—NO, foods should be dense with nutrients.

☒ **Avoid drinking while eating—YES, fluids should be consumed between meals.**

☒ **Restrict total meal size to less than 1 cup—YES, the new stomach pouch only has a capacity of 20 to 30 mL.**

☒ **Avoid concentrated sources of carbohydrates—YES, this may lead to symptoms of dumping syndrome.**

❑ Finish eating meals even if feeling full—NO

Exercise 4-60: *Multiple-choice question*

In order to avoid dumping syndrome, which sometimes occurs after gastric surgery, the nurse should teach the patient the following prevention strategies, with the exception of:

A. Meals should contain more dry items than liquid—NO

B. Fluid intake with meals is discouraged—NO, this causes the stomach contents to empty rapidly.

C. Remain in a low Fowler's position for 20 to 30 minutes after meals—NO, this delays stomach emptying.

D. **Decrease fat intake and increase intake of concentrated carbohydrates—YES, fat can be eaten as tolerated, but concentrated carbohydrates can cause symptoms of dumping syndrome.**

Exercise 4-61: *Fill-in*

Considering Sarah's chief complaints and her history of travel outside the United States to a developing country, what is her likely diagnosis? **Viral hepatitis**

Exercise 4-62: *Fill-in*

The causative organism associated with Sarah's disease process is likely the **hepatitis A virus (HAV)** and the incubation period is **14 to 50 days**.

Exercise 4-63: *Fill-in*

Hepatitis A is transmitted primarily through the **fecal–oral** route by ingesting **food** or **fluids** contaminated with the virus.

Exercise 4-64: *Select all that apply*

Identify other ways in which hepatitis A can be transmitted:

❏ Transfusion of blood products—NO, this is more likely to occur with hepatitis B or C.

☒ **Infected food handlers—YES**

☒ **Oral–anal contact during sexual activity—YES**

❏ Needle sticks—NO, this is more likely to occur with hepatitis B or C.

☒ **Poor hygiene—YES, particularly in day care centers and institutions with clients with developmental disabilities.**

☒ **Consuming raw shellfish—YES, if waters are contaminated with sewage.**

Exercise 4-65: *Select all that apply*

Identify other clinical manifestations associated with hepatitis A:

☒ **Fatigue—YES**

❏ Rashes—NO, may occur with hepatitis B.

☒ **Anorexia—YES, often occurs early and may be severe.**

❏ Ascites—NO

☒ **Dark urine—YES, this occurs associated with jaundice.**

☒ **Aversion to strong odors—YES, an example would be cigarette smoke.**

Exercise 4-66: *True or false*
Identify whether the following statements about the management of hepatitis A are true or false:

__True__ 1. Early studies have shown that a high-protein, high-calorie diet may be beneficial in managing viral hepatitis.

__True__ 2. Alcohol should be avoided during the acute illness and for 6 months after recovery.

__True__ 3. Good personal hygiene and hand washing are important in preventing the spread of hepatitis to family members.

__False__ 4. The hepatitis A vaccine should be given after the acute infection of hepatitis A is past

Exercise 4-67: *Multiple-choice question*
After educating Sarah about the effects that hepatitis has on the liver, the nurse determines that she understands the information when she states:

A. "It is okay to use acetaminophen (Tylenol) as much as needed for aches and pains."—NO, Tylenol is a medication that should be avoided while the liver is inflamed.

B. "I should talk to my physician before taking any herbal or over-the-counter medications."—YES, some herbal products affect the liver and should not be used during acute hepatitis or the recovery period.

C. "Hepatitis causes very little damage to my liver, so I can start taking more vitamin supplements."—NO, hepatitis is damaging to the liver so during the acute and recovery periods of hepatitis, it is not recommended to start taking new supplements.

D. "I will only have one drink on the weekends when I go out with my friends."—NO, alcohol is toxic to the liver and should be avoided during the acute phase of hepatitis and for 6 months after recovery.

Exercise 4-68: *Fill-in*
Briefly explain the effect that an elevated bilirubin level has on the body:
When the concentration of bilirubin in the blood is abnormally elevated, the body tissues become stained yellow or green-yellow; this is called jaundice. Jaundice is evident when the bilirubin level is greater than 2.5 mg/dL.

Exercise 4-69: *Matching*
Match the type of jaundice in Column A with its cause in Column B.

Column A	Column B
A. Hemolytic jaundice	__C__ Extrahepatic obstruction (gallstones)
B. Hepatocellular jaundice	__A__ Increased destruction of erythrocytes
C. Obstructive jaundice	__D__ Inherited disorder
D. Hereditary hyperbilirubinemia	__B__ Damaged liver cells unable to clear bilirubin normally

Exercise 4-70: *Fill-in*

Sarah is likely experiencing **hepatocellular** jaundice related to liver damage caused by the hepatitis A virus.

Exercise 4-71: *Select all that apply*

Identify situations/populations where the hepatitis A vaccine may be recommended:

☒ **Travel to areas with questionable/poor sanitation—YES**

☒ **Homosexual men—YES**

❑ Dialysis patients—NO, this population is more at risk for hepatitis B.

❑ Hemophiliacs—NO, this population is more at risk for hepatitis B.

☒ **Staff of day care centers—YES**

☒ **Health care personnel—YES**

Exercise 4-72: *Fill-in*

Identify the recommended dosing schedule for the hepatitis A vaccines:

1. Adults **two doses total—Give second dose 6 to 12 months after the first.**
2. Children/adolescents 2 to 18 years of age **three doses total—Give second dose 1 month after the first and then give the third dose 6 to 12 months later.**

Exercise 4-73: *Fill-in*

Briefly explain how people who are exposed to hepatitis A, but have never been vaccinated, are treated:

Hepatitis A can be prevented if immune globulin is administered within 2 weeks of exposure. Antibody production is increased, and the person has 6 to 8 weeks of passive immunity. If hepatitis A develops, it is usually a mild case, which then confers immunity against future exposures to hepatitis A.

Exercise 4-74: *Matching*

Match the type of cirrhosis in Column A with its cause in Column B.

Column A	Column B
A. Alcoholic cirrhosis	__B__ Late result of acute viral hepatitis
B. Postnecrotic cirrhosis	__C__ Results from chronic biliary obstruction
C. Biliary cirrhosis	__A__ Results from chronic alcoholism

Exercise 4-75: *Fill-in*

The major causative factor of fatty liver and cirrhosis is **excessive alcohol consumption,** although **malnutrition with reduced protein intake** also contributes to liver destruction.

Exercise 4-76: *Fill-in*
Briefly explain why cirrhotic livers are described as having a hobnail appearance:
The disease progression of cirrhosis is characterized by episodes of necrosis and regeneration of liver cells. Eventually, damaged liver cells are replaced by scar tissue. The hobnail appearance is a result of scar tissue and residual normal or regenerating tissue throughout the liver.

Exercise 4-77: *Select all that apply*
Identify signs and symptoms associated with compensated cirrhosis:

❑ Hypotension—NO, this occurs with decompensated cirrhosis.

☒ **Palmar erythema—YES**

☒ **Vascular spiders—YES**

☒ **Vague morning indigestion—YES**

❑ Jaundice—NO, this occurs with decompensated cirrhosis.

❑ Ascites—NO, this occurs with decompensated cirrhosis.

Exercise 4-78: *Fill-in*
Identify five functions of the liver:
  1. **Glucose metabolism**
  2. **Ammonia conversion**
  3. **Protein metabolism**
  4. **Fat metabolism**
  5. **Vitamin and iron storage**
  6. **Bile formation**
  7. **Bilirubin excretion**
  8. **Drug metabolism**

Exercise 4-79: *Select all that apply*
Identify clinical manifestations associated with ascites:

☒ **Increased abdominal girth—YES, a large amount of albumin-rich fluid accumulates in the abdomen.**

❑ Hematemesis—NO

☒ **Rapid weight gain—YES, related to sodium and water retention by the kidney.**

☒ **Distended veins on abdominal wall—YES**

☒ **Shortness of breath—YES, if abdomen is significantly distended.**

❑ Asterixis—NO, this is associated with hepatic encephalopathy.

Exercise 4-80: *Select all that apply*
Identify clinical manifestations associated with hepatic encephalopathy:

❏ Melena—NO

☒ **Change in mood and sleep patterns—YES**

☒ **Constructional apraxia—YES, this is the inability to draw a simple figure.**

☒ **Fetor hepaticus—YES, this breath odor is described as sweet, slightly fecal.**

❏ Hypotension—NO

☒ **Asterixis—YES, this is a flapping of the hands.**

Exercise 4-81: *True or false*
Identify whether the following statements about ascites and hepatic encephalopathy are true or false:

__True__ 1. The presence of fluid in the abdomen (ascites) can be confirmed by assessing for a fluid wave or percussing for shifting dullness.

__True__ 2. In stage 4 of hepatic encephalopathy, patients are comatose with markedly abnormal electroencephalograms.

__False__ 3. Furosemide (Lasix), an aldosterone-blocking agent, is first-line therapy in the treatment of ascites.

__True__ 4. Some restriction of protein is usually needed in patients who are comatose or have encephalopathy.

Exercise 4-82: *Multiple-choice question*
When Bob's wife asks why he is on a 2-g sodium, protein-restricted diet, the nurse's best response is:

A. "That is not important right now; he will not go home on this diet."—NO, he will likely be discharged on a 2-g sodium diet with some protein restriction.

B. "The salt and protein restriction will allow his liver to heal."—NO, the diet helps with his symptoms, but will not heal the liver.

C. **"The restrictions reduce fluid retention and ammonia levels, thus improving his symptoms."—YES, the restricted sodium reduces fluid retention and the restricted protein reduces ammonia levels.**

D. "This diet is prescribed to help him lose some weight."—NO, the patient will likely lose weight related to less fluid retention, but this is not the purpose of the diet.

Exercise 4-83: *Select all that apply*
Identify causes of increased ammonia levels in patients with hepatic cirrhosis:

❏ Antibiotic administration—NO, neomycin sulfate may decrease ammonia levels.

☒ **Gastrointestinal bleeding—YES, from breakdown of blood proteins.**

☒ **High-protein diets—YES, the breakdown of protein produces ammonia.**

❏ Hyperkalemia—NO, hypokalemia increases the ammonia absorbed from the gastrointestinal tract.

☒ **Bacterial infections—YES, bacteria produce ammonia.**

❑ Acidosis—NO, alkalosis increases the ammonia absorbed from the gastrointestinal tract.

Exercise 4-84: *Multiple-choice question*
After educating Bob's wife about his protein-restricted diet, the nurse determines that she understands the information when she states:
A. "Protein should be eliminated from the diet to prevent increasing ammonia levels."—NO, protein restriction is avoided unless absolutely necessary.
B. "Animal protein is usually better tolerated than vegetable or dairy protein."—NO, usually vegetable protein produces less effect on the ammonia level.
C. "Larger, less frequent meals are more effective in preventing protein loading."—NO, small, frequent meals produce less protein loading.
D. **"Protein intake can be increased if mental status is improving, but should be reduced if neurological signs/symptoms return."—YES, usually 1.0 to 1.5 g/ kg/day are tolerated.**

Exercise 4-85: *Fill-in*
Based on Patrick's presenting signs and symptoms, it is likely that he is having a problem with either **cholecystitis** or **cholelithiasis**.

Exercise 4-86: *Fill-in*
Briefly explain how the gallbladder functions and delivers bile to the duodenum:
Between meals, bile produced by the hepatocytes of the liver enters the gallbladder for storage. When food enters the duodenum, the gallbladder contracts and delivers bile through the cystic and common bile duct to the duodenum.

Exercise 4-87: *Fill-in*
Briefly explain the difference between cholecystitis and cholelithiasis:
Cholecystitis is an acute inflammation of the gallbladder that can occur as a result of a stone obstructing bile outflow, or in less than 10% of cases, it can occur in the absence of obstruction. Cholelithiasis is when cholesterol or pigment calculi form in the gallbladder from solid constituents of bile.

Exercise 4-88: *Select all that apply*
Identify common risk factors for cholelithiasis:
☒ **Obesity—YES**

❑ Male gender—NO, occurs two to three times more frequently in women.

❑ High fat diets—NO

☒ **Rapid weight loss—YES, plus frequent weight changes lead to rapid development of stones.**

☒ **Diabetes mellitus—YES**

❑ Age less than 40—NO, risk increases with age; more common after 40 years of age.

Exercise 4-89: *Select all that apply*
Identify clinical manifestations associated with cholelithiasis:

☒ **Biliary colic—YES, this is a severe right upper quadrant pain that radiates to the back or right shoulder and is associated with nausea and vomiting.**

☒ **Jaundice—YES, if the common bile duct is obstructed.**

☒ **Change in urine and stool color—YES, this occurs with obstruction and increased renal excretion of bile pigments.**

❑ Melena—NO

❑ Diarrhea—NO

☒ **Pruritus—YES, if jaundice is present.**

Exercise 4-90: *Calculation*
Order: hydromorphone (Dilaudid) 1.5 mg IV every 3 hours PRN
   Dilaudid is supplied as 2 mg in 1 mL.
Calculate the dose of Dilaudid to be given in mL: __0.75 mL__

Exercise 4-91: *True or false*
Identify whether the following statements about the medical management of cholelithiasis are true or false:

__True__ 1. Nonsurgical treatments provide only a temporary solution and are associated with persistent symptoms and recurrent stone formation.

__False__ 2. Ursodeoxycholic acid is effective in dissolving or reducing the size of pigment stones.

__False__ 3. Extracorporeal shock wave lithotripsy, which uses shock waves to break up stones, is the treatment of choice for gallbladder disease.

__True__ 4. Laparoscopic cholecystectomies have decreased the surgical risks, length of hospital stay, and recovery period compared to the open cholecystectomies.

Exercise 4-92: *Select all that apply*
Identify foods that should be avoided in patients who have intolerances to fatty foods and vague gastrointestinal symptoms associated with biliary disease:

❑ Skim milk—NO

❑ Mashed potatoes—NO

☒ **Fried foods—YES, this may induce an episode of cholecystitis.**

☒ **Cheese—YES, this may induce an episode of cholecystitis.**

❑ Bread—NO

☒ **Alcohol—YES, this may induce an episode of cholecystitis.**

Exercise 4-93: *Fill-in*

Identify three potential nursing diagnoses for the patient postoperatively following gallbladder surgery:

1. **Acute pain and discomfort related to surgical incision**
2. **Imbalanced nutrition, less than body requirements, related to inadequate bile secretion**
3. **Deficient knowledge related to self-care activities (incision care, diet modification, potential complications)**
4. **Risk for infection related to surgical incision**

Exercise 4-94: *Multiple-choice question*

When Patrick's wife asks why he is having pain in his right shoulder, the nurse's best response is:

A. "The pain is related to how he was positioned during surgery."—NO

B. "This pain may indicate that he still has a stone lodged somewhere."—NO

C. "This pain is referred from the site where his gallbladder was removed."—NO

D. **"Pain occurs in this location from the gas used to inflate the abdomen during surgery."—YES, carbon dioxide is infused into the abdominal cavity with laparoscopic surgeries to allow for visualization of the abdominal organs.**

Exercise 4-95: *Fill-in*

Briefly explain why patients are placed on a low-fat diet following surgery:

It takes 4 to 6 weeks for the biliary ducts to dilate to compensate for the amount of bile previously stored by the gallbladder. After this time frame, when fats are eaten, an adequate amount of bile will be released to emulsify the fats and assist with digestion.

Exercise 4-96: *Multiple-choice question*

After educating Patrick about his activity restrictions after discharge, the nurse determines that he understands the information when he states:

A. "I should do nothing but rest the next couple of weeks."—NO, he can begin light exercise, like walking, immediately.

B. "I should avoid showering the next 3 days."—NO, he can shower when 1 to 2 days postoperative.

C. **"I need to wait 3 to 4 days before driving."—YES**

D. "I can't wait to pick up and hug my 4-year-old when I get home."—NO, he should avoid lifting over 5 pounds for the next week.

Exercise 4-97: *Multiple-choice question*

As Patrick asks further questions about wound care, the nurse determines that he needs further instruction when he states:

A. "I need to call the physician if I have a fever or notice redness or drainage at the site.—NO

B. "I should change these Steri-Strips daily and apply new dressings."—YES, Steri-Strips should be allowed to fall off on their own; dressings are not needed.

C. "These wounds can be washed with soap and water."—NO

D. "I can leave these wounds open to air."—NO

Exercise 4-98: *Fill-in*

Based on Roy's presenting signs and symptoms and his significant alcohol history, it is possible that Roy has **acute pancreatitis**.

Exercise 4-99: *Fill-in*

Identify three digestive enzymes secreted by the exocrine pancreas and their function:

1. **Amylase—aids in digestion of carbohydrates**
2. **Trypsin—aids in digestion of proteins**
3. **Lipase—aids in digestion of fats**

Exercise 4-100: *Select all that apply*

Identify clinical manifestations associated with acute pancreatitis:

☒ **Acute, severe abdominal pain that occurs 24 to 48 hours after a heavy meal or alcohol intake—YES, and it is unrelieved by antacids.**

☐ Hypercalcemia—NO, hypocalcemia occurs with loss of protein-rich fluid into the peritoneal cavity.

☒ **Nausea unrelieved by vomiting—YES**

☐ Hypervolemia—NO, hypovolemia occurs with loss of protein-rich fluid into the peritoneal cavity.

☒ **Ecchymosis in the flank or umbilical area—YES, if pancreatitis is severe.**

☒ **Abdominal guarding—YES**

Exercise 4-101: *Fill-in*

Identify why the above laboratory tests are abnormal related to the diagnosis of acute pancreatitis:

1. Amylase: **Indicates a pancreatic problem; elevates within 24 hours of symptom onset**
2. Lipase: **Indicates a pancreatic problem; elevates within 24 hours of symptom onset**
3. White blood cells: **Elevates with inflammation associated with acute pancreatitis**
4. Glucose: **Elevates because pancreatic inflammation can interfere with normal endocrine function**
5. Calcium: **Decreases because of loss of protein-rich fluid into peritoneal cavity**

Exercise 4-102: *Multiple-choice question*
When Roy's wife asks how acute pancreatitis develops, the nurse's best response is:

A. **"Acute pancreatitis is autodigestion of the pancreas by its own enzymes; it occurs most often with gallstones or long-term alcohol use."—YES, in 80% of patients.**

B. "Acute pancreatitis is most often caused by tumors of the pancreas or intestines."—NO

C. "Acute pancreatitis occurs when the pancreas is damaged by frequently eating spicy, hot foods combined with alcohol."—NO, symptoms may occur after a heavy meal, but it doesn't specifically develop as a result of eating spicy food.

D. "Acute pancreatitis occurs in patients with hypertension who have blood pressures that are high for prolonged periods."—NO

Exercise 4-103: *Fill-in*
Briefly explain why strict NPO is enforced for patients with pancreatitis:
Oral intake is withheld to inhibit stimulation of the pancreas and release of pancreatic enzymes, which would further cause autodigestion of the pancreas and worsen acute pancreatitis.

Exercise 4-104: *Calculation*
Order: Morphine 2 mg IV every 2 hours PRN
  Morphine is supplied as 5 mg in 2 mL.
Calculate the dose of morphine to be given in mL: **0.8 mL**

Exercise 4-105: *Calculation*
Order: Sliding-scale insulin coverage with lispro (Humalog)
  Formula: For blood sugars > 150 mg/dL: (Blood sugar − 100) divided by 30
  Fingerstick blood sugar is 194.
Calculate the amount of Humalog to be given in units: **3 units**

Exercise 4-106: *True or false*
Identify whether the following statements about the medical management of acute pancreatitis are true or false:
  True 1. Patients with acute pancreatitis require aggressive respiratory care because of the high risk of pulmonary infiltrates, effusions, and atelectasis.
  False 2. Nasogastric tubes are routinely ordered in patients with acute pancreatitis in order to remove gastric secretions.
  True 3. Hypotension and decreased urine output are treated with fluids and blood products to replace fluid lost.
  True 4. After recovery from acute pancreatitis, patients are advised to avoid high-fat foods, heavy meals, and alcohol.

Exercise 4-107: *Multiple-choice question*

After educating Roy and his wife about the need to turn and reposition every 2 hours, the nurse determines that the wife understands the information when she states:

A. "Turning every 2 hours will help to reduce the pain he is feeling."—NO, this will not reduce pain levels.

B. "Getting out of bed and walking is actually the best for him."—NO, bed rest is required to reduce pancreatic and gastric secretions.

C. **"Frequent position changes help prevent skin breakdown and lung problems."—YES**

D. "Keeping him flat in bed will help him to breath better."—NO, a semi-Fowler's position will promote increased respiratory expansion.

Exercise 4-108: *Multiple-choice question*

When Roy's wife asks how patient-controlled analgesia (PCA) works, the nurse's best response is:

A. "The patient or family can push the button at any time to deliver pain medication."—NO, families are discouraged from pushing the button, especially when patients are sleeping, because this overrides one of the system's safety features.

B. **"PCA pumps allow patients to control administration of their medication, often resulting in better pain relief."—YES**

C. "PCA pumps improve pain control, but greatly increase the risk of overdose."—NO, safety features are in place, but patients still require respiratory assessment.

D. "The family needs to ensure the patient is breathing well before the button is pushed."—NO, it is the nurse's responsibility to assess the patient.

5

Nursing Care of the Patient With Neurological Disease

Karen K. Gittings

Unfolding Case Study #30 ▪ Austin

Austin is a 19-year-old college student with a history of epilepsy since childhood; the cause of his seizures have never been identified. His epilepsy has been well controlled on phenytoin (Dilantin). Today while walking to classes, Austin falls to the ground seizing. His friends call for an ambulance, and Austin is brought into the emergency department (ED). On arrival, Austin is drowsy and confused. Two of his friends arrive in the ED shortly after.

Exercise 5-1: *Fill-in*
Since the cause of Austin's seizures is unknown, he would be classified as having _____ epilepsy.

Exercise 5-2: *Select all that apply*
Identify other potential causes of seizures:

❑ Diabetes

❑ Head injuries

❑ Fever

❑ Lung cancer

❑ Brain tumors

❑ Central nervous system infections

❑ Excessive smoking

ⓔ **eResource 5-1:** To learn more about the causes of seizures, consult the Merck Manual: [Pathway: www.merckmanuals.com → select "Merck Manual of Diagnosis and Therapy" → enter "seizure disorder" into the search field and review content regarding etiology. Don't forget to look at the table of causes]

The nurse questions Austin's friends about what happened before, during, and after the seizure. The friends reported that they were just walking to class when Austin fell to the ground, became very stiff, and his arms and legs began convulsing. They tried to hold him so that he would not hurt himself. They also noticed that his mouth was clamped shut, and he had saliva coming from the corner. After the seizure stopped, Austin was breathing heavily, and they saw blood in his mouth.

Exercise 5-3: *Fill-in*

Based upon the information provided by Austin's friends, this would be classified as a
_____ seizure.

Exercise 5-4: *Fill-in*

Briefly explain the pathophysiology underlying seizures:

_____

_____

_____

_____

Exercise 5-5: *Select all that apply*

Identify clinical manifestations associated with generalized seizures:

❑ Epileptic cry

❑ Tonic-clonic contraction

❑ Unintelligible speech

❑ Excessive emotions

❑ Incontinence of urine or stool

❑ Tongue biting

Austin is more alert and asking questions about what happened. The nurse orients him to his environment and explains that he had a seizure; Austin does not remember events leading up to it or whether or not he had an aura. When the nurse questions him about his medications, Austin reports that he is on phenytoin (Dilantin) 200 mg orally twice a day, but he ran out of his medication 2 days ago. The provider orders a Dilantin level.

 eResource 5-2: To verify the therapeutic serum level for Dilantin, refer to Epocrates on your mobile device: [Pathway: Epocrates → enter "Dilantin" into the search field → scroll down to "Safety/Monitoring" to review content]

Answers to this chapter begin on page 197.

Exercise 5-6: *Fill-in*

An aura is a_____, _____, or_____
premonitory or warning sensation.

Exercise 5-7: *Select all that apply*

Identify the most common side effects associated with chronic phenytoin (Dilantin) use:

- ❏ Aplastic anemia
- ❏ Gingival hyperplasia
- ❏ Nausea
- ❏ Nystagmus
- ❏ Agranulocytosis
- ❏ Hirsutism

ⓔ **eResource 5-3:** To reinforce your understanding of common side effects associated with Dilantin, refer to Epocrates on your mobile device: [Pathway: Epocrates → enter "Dilantin" into the search field → scroll down to "Common Reactions" and review content]

Exercise 5-8: *Matching*

Match the generic anticonvulsant medication in Column A with its trade name in Column B.

Column A	Column B
A. carbamazepine	_____ Keppra
B. clonazepam	_____ Neurontin
C. gabapentin	_____ Tegretol
D. levetiracetam	_____ Depakote
E. valproate	_____ Klonopin

ⓔ **eResource 5-4:** To reinforce your understanding and to learn more about anticonvulsant medications, refer to Medscape on your mobile device: [Pathway: Medscape → enter "Epilepsy" into the search field → select "Epilepsy and Seizures" → select "Medication" tab → select "Anticonvulsant Agents" and review content]

Austin's parents have arrived at the hospital. They are very concerned that Austin did not tell them that he ran out of his medication. They are informed that his low Dilantin level likely led to his seizure. Austin is given a dose of phenytoin (Dilantin) and will be discharged shortly. The nurse spends a significant amount of time re-educating Austin and his parents on epilepsy, medication control, and safety concerns.

Answers to this chapter begin on page 197.

eResource 5-5: For supplemental information regarding patient and family teaching, refer to Epocrates Online: [Pathway: http://online. epocrates.com → enter "epilepsy" into the search field → select "Generalized seizures in adults" → review content under "Follow-up" focusing on "Patient Instructions" and "Complications"]

Exercise 5-9: *Fill-in*

Identify three potential nursing diagnoses relevant to the patient with a history of seizures:

1. _____

2. _____

3. _____

Exercise 5-10: *True or false*

Identify whether the following interventions for epilepsy are true or false:

_____ 1. Adhering to the prescribed medication regimen, with periodic monitoring of drug levels, is essential for controlling seizures.

_____ 2. Alcoholic beverages should be avoided because they can increase the risk of seizures.

_____ 3. At home, patients with epilepsy are advised to purchase padded side rails for their beds.

_____ 4. Patients are advised to avoid sleep deprivation, which may lower the seizure threshold.

Exercise 5-11: *Multiple-choice question*

A ketogenic diet, which has been found effective in controlling seizures in children, consists of:

      A. High-protein, high-carbohydrate, low-fat foods

      B. Low-protein, high-carbohydrate, low-fat foods

      C. Low-protein, low-carbohydrate, high-fat foods

      D. High-protein, low-carbohydrate, high-fat foods

Exercise 5-12: *Multiple-choice question*

When Austin's mother asks if there are any other factors that may precipitate a seizure, the nurse's best response is:

      A. "He just needs to take his medication like it is ordered."

      B. "Emotional states, environmental stressors, or fever can trigger a seizure."

      C. "The start of menstruation can cause a seizure to occur."

      D. "He should stop playing video games and watching television because they can precipitate seizures."

Answers to this chapter begin on page 197.

eResource 5-6: For more information about seizure triggers, refer to Merck Manual Online: [Pathway: www.merckmanuals.com → select "Merck Manual of Diagnosis and Therapy" → enter "seizures" into the search field → select "seizure disorders" → review content under "History." Be sure to scroll down to review Tables 1 and 3]

Exercise 5-13: *Select all that apply*

Identify safety-related interventions relevant for the patient with epilepsy:

❏ Educate family and friends about patient care during a seizure

❏ Notify all patient contacts about the patient's diagnosis of epilepsy

❏ Inform all health care providers of medications being taken

❏ Encourage patients to wear a medical information bracelet

Austin is almost ready for discharge. His friends are with him, and they ask what they should do in the future if he has another seizure. The nurse explains appropriate care for the patient having a seizure.

Exercise 5-14: *Multiple-choice question*

After educating Austin's friends about care during a seizure, the nurse determines that they understand the information when one of them states:

    A. "We should protect his head, but not attempt to restrain him."

    B. "We should try to open his mouth so he doesn't bite his tongue."

    C. "We should try to get him in the car to bring him to the hospital."

    D. "We should keep him on his back after the seizure until help arrives."

 eResource 5-7: For more supplemental teaching material for Austin's friends, refer to:

    ■ Medline Plus interactive tutorial, *Seizures & Epilepsy*: http://goo.gl/GWTsG

    ■ Careplans Online to review a nursing care plan for patients with seizure disorders: http://goo.gl/hXyWA

Unfolding Case Study #31   Pam

Pam is a 74-year-old female who was brought to the emergency department (ED) by ambulance after her husband noticed her having difficulty walking and dragging her left leg. She has a history of hypertension, myocardial infarction, peripheral vascular disease, type 2 diabetes, and obesity. Vital signs are obtained, an intravenous (IV) line is inserted, and Pam is quickly sent for a noncontrast computed tomographic (CT) scan. Results from the CT scan reveal that Pam is having an ischemic stroke.

e **eResource 5-8:** To help Pam learn more about this procedure, refer to Medline Plus: [Pathway: www.nlm.nih.gov → select "MedLinePlus" → enter "CT scan" into the search field → select "read more" → select "cranial CT" and review content. Or use quick link: http://goo.gl/bwI6h]

Exercise 5-15: *Select all that apply*

Identify the risk factors for ischemic stroke that are modifiable:

❑ Age

❑ Hypertension

❑ Atrial fibrillation

❑ Hyperlipidemia

❑ Race

❑ Smoking

e **eResource 5-9:** To learn more about risk factors associated with stroke, refer to Epocrates Online: [Pathway: http://online.epocrates.com → select the "diseases" tab → enter "stroke" into the search field → select "risk factors" and review content]

Exercise 5-16: *Fill-in*

Briefly explain the pathophysiology underlying ischemic strokes:

_____

_____

e **eResource 5-10:** To better understand what happens during a stroke, watch the following video, *The Basics of Stroke:* http://youtu.be/xbyfeEW56Nc

Exercise 5-17: *Fill-in*

An ischemic area of brain tissue surrounding the infarcted area, the _____, can be salvaged with timely intervention.

Exercise 5-18: *Select all that apply*

Identify clinical manifestations associated with ischemic strokes:

❑ Hemiplegia or hemiparesis

❑ Confusion or change in mental status

❑ Shortness of breath

❑ Dysphasia or aphasia

❑ Blindness

❑ Sensory loss

❑ Psychological effects

Answers to this chapter begin on page 197.

Exercise 5-19: *Matching*

Match the stroke location in Column A with its common symptoms/behaviors in Column B. Answers in Column A can be used more than once.

Column A	Column B
A. Right hemispheric stroke	_____ Paralysis on left side of body
B. Left hemispheric stroke	_____ Aphasia
	_____ Slow, cautious behavior
	_____ Spatial-perceptual deficits
	_____ Altered intellectual ability
	_____ Impulsive behavior and poor judgment

eResource 5-11: To learn more about the clinical presentation of stroke:
- Consult Medscape: [Pathway: Medscape → enter "stroke" into the search field → select "ischemic stroke" → select "clinical presentation" → select "history" and "physical examination" and review content]
- View the following video depicting the symptoms of Transient Ischemic Attack (TIA) or mini-stroke: http://youtu.be/L7UvhwORTd4

Pam's stroke symptoms are not resolving. Laboratory tests have been ordered and blood has been already drawn and sent. The provider is using a checklist to determine whether Pam is eligible to receive thrombolytic therapy.

Exercise 5-20: *Fill-in*

Identify five contraindications to administering thrombolytic therapy:

1. _____
2. _____
3. _____
4. _____
5. _____

eResource 5-12: To learn more about the contraindications/risks associated with thrombolytic therapy, refer to the Merck Manual: [Pathway: www.merckmanuals.com → select "Merck Manual of Diagnosis and Therapy" → enter "thrombolytic therapy" into the search field → review content]

The provider has determined that Pam is a candidate for thrombolytic therapy with tissue plasminogen activator (t-PA). Two additional IV sites are started for blood draws and other medications. Pam is weighed, and the pharmacy is notified to calculate her t-PA dose based on a weight of 224 pounds. Shortly after her eligibility is determined, Pam begins receiving the t-PA.

Answers to this chapter begin on page 197.

eResource 5-13: To understand the criteria used in determining eligibility for receiving the t-PA, refer to Medscape on your mobile device: [Pathway: Medscape → enter "thrombolytic" into the search field → select "thrombolytic therapy in stroke" → select "thrombolysis guidelines" and review content]

Exercise 5-21: *Calculation*
Order: t-PA dose is 0.9 mg/kg with a maximum dose of 90 mg. Ten percent is to be given IV bolus over 1 minute. The remaining 90% is to be given over 1 hour via infusion pump.

Calculate the total dose of t-PA: _____

Calculate the amount to be administered over 1 minute: _____

Calculate the amount to be administered over 1 hour: _____

 eResource 5-14: To verify your calculations, refer to MedCalc on your mobile device: [Pathway: MedCalc → enter "infusion" into the search field → select "infusion drip rate" → enter infusion order into fields]

Exercise 5-22: *Select all that apply*
Identify factors associated with the occurrence of intracranial bleeding post t-PA:

❑ Age greater than 70 years

❑ Serum glucose 300 mg/dL or greater

❑ Increased calcium levels

❑ Cerebral edema on patient's first CT scan

❑ African American race

❑ Male gender

Pam is transferred to the medical intensive care unit where she is monitored closely. Vital signs are initially monitored every 15 minutes. Neurological checks are done hourly. Pam is assessed frequently for signs of bleeding.

Exercise 5-23: *Fill-in*
Identify three potential nursing diagnoses for the patient diagnosed with an ischemic stroke:

1. _____

2. _____

3. _____

 eResource 5-15: For more information regarding a nursing care plan for Pam, refer to Careplans Online: http://goo.gl/jZsam

Pam has no complications with her thrombolytic therapy. She has residual weakness in her left arm and leg, so arrangements are being made for her transfer to a rehabilitation facility.

Answers to this chapter begin on page 197.

Exercise 5-24: *True or false*

Identify whether the following nursing interventions for care of the stroke patient are true or false:

_____ 1. Unaffected extremities are exercised passively three to four times a day to maintain joint mobility and regain motor control.

_____ 2. Patients are first taught to maintain sitting and standing balance before attempting ambulation.

_____ 3. Instruct patients to carry out self-care activities on the unaffected side.

_____ 4. Health care personnel should assist patients with expressive aphasia by finishing their thoughts or sentences.

Exercise 5-25: *Multiple-choice question*

When Pam's daughter asks why her mother is not receiving as much help as when she was in the hospital, the nurse's best response is:

    A. "We have fewer nurses and patient care technicians than the hospitals."

    B. "She needs to learn to take care of herself now."

    C. "Usually the families help with the patient's care."

    D. "We are trying to help your mother regain as much independence as possible."

Exercise 5-26: *Fill-in*

Identify five assistive devices designed to improve the self-care of stroke patients:

1. _____

2. _____

3. _____

4. _____

5. _____

 eResource 5-16: For more information regarding stroke rehabilitation resources, refer to:
- NIH's *Post-Stroke Rehabilitation Fact Sheet*: http://goo.gl/92Pz4
- Department of Veterans Affairs, *Stroke Rehabilitation*: http://goo.gl/ruARI
- MedLinePlus's interactive tutorial, *Stroke Rehabilitation*: http://goo.gl/7ES7Z

Exercise 5-27: *Multiple-choice question*

After talking to Pam's husband and daughter about the potential effects of caregiving on the family, the nurse determines that the daughter understands the information when she states:

    A. "Dad needs to take on all of mom's responsibilities now."

    B. "Dad needs to remain close to mom at all times while at home."

Answers to this chapter begin on page 197.

C. "Mom is going to initially need 24-hour supervision, so we need to plan ways to give dad a break."

D. "Dad has always looked out for mom, so he will have no trouble taking her home."

Pam is soon discharged to the care of her family. She has made great progress and will continue her rehabilitation as an outpatient.

 eResource 5-17: For more information regarding recommended follow-up following a stroke, consult Epocrates Online: [Pathway: http://online.epocrates.com → select the "diseases" tab → enter "stroke" → select "Ischemic stroke" → select "Follow-up" and review content]

Unfolding Case Study #32 ▬ Dean

Dean is a 23-year-old male brought to the emergency department following a motor vehicle accident. The accident occurred while he was on the job driving a company van; he was unrestrained and found in the passenger side of the van. He was brought in on a backboard with a neck collar in place. Dean is awake and alert; he states that he is unable to feel his legs. The trauma team is mobilized, and the provider is currently assessing Dean.

Exercise 5-28: *Select all that apply*
Identify risk factors for spinal cord injuries:

❑ Young age

❑ Alcohol use

❑ Smoking

❑ African American race

❑ Drug use

❑ Male gender

Exercise 5-29: *Ordering*
Rank the causes of spinal cord injuries in order of their frequency of occurrence:

_____ Recreational sporting activities

_____ Falls

_____ Violence (gunshot wounds)

_____ Motor vehicle accidents

 eResource 5-18: To learn more about the causes of spinal cord injuries, consult Medscape on your mobile device: [Pathway: Medscape → enter → "spinal cord" into the search field → select "spinal cord injuries" → under the "overview" section, review "epidemiology"]

Answers to this chapter begin on page 197.

eResource 5-19: To learn more about spinal cord injuries, view the following videos:
- *Basic Facts about Spinal Cord Injuries:* http://youtu.be/6jpQhStDX9M
- *Levels of Function in Spinal Cord Injury:* http://youtu.be/PseUxltIw_U

Dean complains of acute pain in his upper back area and chest. He is heard to say, "I think I broke my back." The provider completes his neurological examination. Dean has no sensation or motor function below the level of T5. X-rays and a CT scan are ordered. Dean is kept immobilized on the backboard with the neck collar in place.

 eResource 5-20: To learn more about the recommended diagnostic work-up, including x-rays and CT scan, continue reading in Medscape: [Pathway: Medscape → enter "spinal cord" into the search field → select "spinal cord injuries" → select the "Workup" tab and review content]

Exercise 5-30: *Multiple-choice question*
In order to prevent further damage when moving a patient with a potential spinal cord injury, it is important to:
- A. Place the patient in a side-lying position for transport.
- B. Place the patient in traction shortly after arrival in the emergency department.
- C. Avoid all radiographic exams until the injury has been ruled out by neurological examination.
- D. Keep the patient immobilized on a backboard with the head and neck maintained in a neutral position.

The CT scan confirms that Dean has a spinal cord injury at the level of T4–T5. He also has multiple rib fractures and a right femur fracture. Numerous contusions are noted on physical exam. A CT scan of the head is negative. There is no cervical spine injury. The provider has written orders for methylprednisolone 30 mg/kg IV to be given over 15 minutes and then followed 45 minutes later by a continuous infusion of 5.4 mg/kg/hour for 23 hours.

Exercise 5-31: *Calculation*
Order: methylprednisolone 30 mg/kg IV over 15 minutes

     Patient's weight is 198 pounds

Calculate the dose of methylprednisolone: _____

 eResource 5-21: To verify your calculations, refer to MedCalc on your mobile device: [Pathway: MedCalc → enter "infusion" into the search field → select "infusion management" and enter patient data]

Dean is admitted to the trauma-surgical intensive care unit where he will be monitored for signs of acute complications. His parents are now at his bedside. The neurosurgeon has informed Dean and his parents that Dean will need surgery to stabilize his vertebral fractures and femur fracture, but he wants to wait 24 hours.

Answers to this chapter begin on page 197.

Exercise 5-32: *Select all that apply*

Identify acute complications that can occur after a spinal cord injury:

❑ Myocardial infarction

❑ Neurogenic shock

❑ Deep vein thrombosis

❑ Respiratory complications

❑ Stroke

❑ Autonomic dysreflexia

e **eResource 5-22:** To learn more about complications associated with spinal cord injuries, refer to the Merck Manual: [Pathway: www.merckmanuals.com → select "Merck Manual of Diagnosis and Therapy" → enter "spinal cord injury" into the search field → select "spinal cord injury" → select "complications" and review content]

Exercise 5-33: *Fill-in*

Identify five potential nursing diagnoses for the patient diagnosed with acute spinal cord injury:

1. _____

2. _____

3. _____

4. _____

5. _____

e **eResource 5-23:** For supplemental information regarding developing a nursing careplan for Dean, refer to Careplans Online: http://goo.gl/nCBR2

Exercise 5-34: *True or false*

Identify whether the following nursing interventions for the patient with a spinal cord injury are true or false:

_____ 1. Breathing exercises are encouraged for strengthening of inspiratory muscles.

_____ 2. Passive range-of-motion is discouraged below the level of spinal cord injury.

_____ 3. Vigorous suctioning should be used frequently to prevent retention of secretions.

_____ 4. Splints, which are used to prevent footdrop, should be removed and reapplied every 2 hours.

Dean has surgery to stabilize his vertebral and femur fractures. Postoperatively, his vital signs are stable. The provider has written orders to start getting Dean out of bed on the day after surgery. The case manager has been consulted to begin investigating rehabilitation facilities that specialize in treating patients with spinal cord injury.

Answers to this chapter begin on page 197.

Exercise 5-35: *Multiple-choice question*

When Dean's mother asks what can be done to keep his skin in good condition, the nurse's best response is:

    A. "Unfortunately, it is inevitable that he will develop skin breakdown at some point."

    B. "Most importantly, we need to turn and reposition him at least every 2 hours."

    C. "Using lotion once a day will keep his skin smooth and soft."

    D. "They will teach you that information before he leaves the rehabilitation facility."

 eResource 5-24: To provide additional teaching for Dean's mother, refer to University of Washington Medical Center's patient pamphlets regarding *Maintaining Health Skin*:
- Part 1: http://goo.gl/77Eij
- Part 2: http://goo.gl/5tV3h

Exercise 5-36: *Multiple-choice question*

Patients are initially allowed nothing by mouth (NPO) after a spinal cord injury, but once bowel sounds return, they should begin a diet that is:

    A. High-calorie, high-protein, high-fiber

    B. Low-calorie, high-protein, low-fiber

    C. Low-calorie, high-protein, high-fiber

    D. High-calorie, high-protein, low-fiber

Exercise 5-37: *Select all that apply*

Identify interventions designed to minimize the risk of thrombophlebitis in the patient with an acute spinal cord injury:

    ❏ Anticoagulation

    ❏ Abdominal binders

    ❏ Antiembolism stockings

    ❏ Adequate hydration

    ❏ Antiplatelet medications

    ❏ Pneumatic compression devices

eResource 5-25: To learn more about the causes of thrombophlebitis and preventive measures, refer to the Merck Manual: [Pathway: www.merckmanuals.com → select "Merck Manual of Diagnosis and Therapy" → enter "thrombophlebitis" into the search field → select "Deep Venous Thrombosis (DVT)" → select "Prevention" and review content]

Exercise 5-38: *Multiple-choice question*
When Dean is heard telling a friend that he will never be anything but a burden for his family, the nurse's best response is:

    A. "Your family loves you and will take good care of you."
    B. "You should be thinking more positive thoughts."
    C. "In rehabilitation, they will be teaching you how to care for yourself."
    D. "Unfortunately, you will always have to live with your family."

Dean is eventually moved to a rehabilitation facility that specializes in spinal cord injuries. He has hope that he will become increasingly independent. His family remains supportive and involved in his care.

 eResource 5-26: For more information to supplement discharge teaching for spinal cord injury, refer to:
    ■ NIH's *Spinal Cord Injury Information Page*: http://goo.gl/0cI9c
    ■ MedLinePlus's interactive tutorial, *Spinal Cord Injury*: http://goo.gl/42IDm

Unfolding Case Study #33 ▨ Kacey

Kacey is a 21-year-old nursing student who saw her primary care provider (PCP) a week ago for complaints of fatigue, weakness, and poor coordination. A magnetic resonance imaging (MRI) scan of the head was ordered by the PCP, and Kacey was instructed what to expect from the procedure.

eResource 5-27: To prepare Kacey for the MRI, the nurse reviewed the following content provided by MedlinePlus: http://goo.gl/2ej6K

Kacey is now back in her PCP's office to learn the results. She is accompanied by her mother. The PCP proceeds to tell Kacey that she has multiple sclerosis.

eResource 5-28: To review the six-step protocol for giving bad news, view *How Best to Deliver Bad News to Patients and Family*: http://youtu.be/ItC68Pdnpk4

eResource 5-29: For a review of Therapeutic Communication view:
    ■ Therapeutic Communication in Psychiatric Nursing: http://goo.gl/UnCdX
    ■ List of Communication Techniques: http://goo.gl/LSgMJ

Exercise 5-39: *Fill-in*
Briefly explain the pathophysiology underlying multiple sclerosis:

_____

_____

eResource 5-30: To better understand the pathophysiology of multiple sclerosis, refer to Medscape: [Pathway: Medscape → enter "Multiple Sclerosis" into the search field → review content under "pathophysiology" also be sure to review the content under the "Workup" tab—particularly the information under "Magnetic Resonance Imaging"]

Exercise 5-40: *Select all that apply*
Identify other clinical manifestations associated with multiple sclerosis:

❏ Depression

❏ Numbness

❏ Dizziness

❏ Visual disturbances

❏ Loss of balance

❏ Pain

❏ Diarrhea

❏ Cognitive changes

(e) **eResource 5-31:** To learn more about the clinical presentation of persons with multiple sclerosis, review the following:
■ Merck Manual: [Pathway: www.merckmanuals.com → select "Merck Manual of Diagnosis and Therapy" → enter "multiple sclerosis" into the search field → select "multiple sclerosis" → select "Symptoms and Signs" and review content]
■ A video describing the early symptoms of multiple sclerosis: http://youtu.be/shG0moR0Hec

Exercise 5-41: *Multiple-choice question*
On MRI, patients with multiple sclerosis have:

A. Increased cerebral spinal fluid

B. Atrophy of gray matter

C. Multiple plaques throughout the central nervous system

D. Inflammation of the basal ganglia

The PCP orders glatiramer (Copaxone) 20 mg subcutaneously daily. The nurse educates Kacey and her mother on correct administration of the drug. They also discuss strategies for dealing with the fatigue.

Exercise 5-42: *Fill-in*
Identify five potential side effects that may occur with administration of glatiramer (Copaxone):

1. _____

2. _____

3. _____

4. _____

5. _____

Answers to this chapter begin on page 197.

eResource 5-32: To reinforce your understanding of the side effects associated with glatiramer, refer to Skyscape's RxDrugs on your mobile device: [Pathway: RxDrugs → enter "glatiramer" into the search field → scroll down to "Adverse Reactions" and review content]

Exercise 5-43: *Ordering*

Number in order the steps required for administration of glatiramer (Copaxone):

_____ Choose injection site in arms, thigh, or abdomen

_____ Discard needle in puncture-resistant container

_____ Allow prefilled syringe to warm to room temperature for 20 minutes

_____ Pinch skin and inject at a 90-degree angle

_____ Inspect medication to ensure it is clear and colorless to slightly yellow

_____ Clean site with alcohol and allow to dry

Exercise 5-44: *True or false*

Identify whether the following strategies for controlling fatigue associated with multiple sclerosis are true or false:

_____ 1. Avoid cold environments and temperatures

_____ 2. Achieve a balance between rest and activities

_____ 3. Stop all medications when fatigue becomes severe

_____ 4. Maintain a healthy lifestyle, avoiding alcohol and smoking

 eResource 5-33: To help Kacey and her mother learn more about managing multiple sclerosis, the nurse shows them a series of videos, *Living Well: A Guide to Managing Multiple Sclerosis:*
- Part 1: http://youtu.be/FD5YoTCQ4W4
- Part 2: http://youtu.be/sTw7w6s6Yhw
- Part 3: http://youtu.be/p6Hk7SqaC_s

Exercise 5-45: *Fill-in*

Identify three potential nursing diagnoses for the patient diagnosed with multiple sclerosis:

1. _____

2. _____

3. _____

 eResource 5-34: For supplemental information to help in the development of a care plan for Kacey, go to Careplans Online: http://goo.gl/gDj24

When Kacey and her mother return home, they begin researching multiple sclerosis on the Internet. They do extensive reading on the disease process and available treatments.

Answers to this chapter begin on page 197.

Exercise 5-46: *Select all that apply*

Identify interventions designed to promote physical mobility in the patient with multiple sclerosis:

❑ Strenuous activity to the point of fatigue

❑ Frequent, short rest periods

❑ Daily exercises for muscle stretching

❑ Exercise in a warm environment

❑ Walking

❑ Hot baths with spasms

Exercise 5-47: *Multiple-choice question*

If difficulty in coordination occurs as a result of motor dysfunction, it is first recommended to:

A. Watch the feet while walking

B. Use an assistive device, such as braces

C. Use a wheelchair or motorized scooter

D. Walk with feet apart to widen the base of support

Kacey and her mother are back to see the PCP for follow-up. Kacey is tolerating the glatiramer (Copaxone) with minimal side effects. Her coordination has improved, although she remains fatigued. In private, Kacey's mother tells the nurse that Kacey is very moody and difficult at times.

Exercise 5-48: *Multiple-choice question*

When Kacey's mother asks what she can do about Kacey's moodiness, the nurse's best response is:

A. "You need to set limits on her behavior."

B. "Just ignore her and she will quit acting out so much."

C. "Suggest that she stay in her room until she is in a better mood."

D. "People adapt to illness differently; support of family and friends is of primary importance."

Kacey is continuing to learn how to successfully manage her disease while continuing with her nursing education.

Unfolding Case Study #34 ▨ Rick

Rick is a 56-year-old male who was diagnosed with Parkinson's disease 3 years ago. He is seeing his primary care provider (PCP) for a routine appointment, and he is accompanied by his wife. He has a medical history of hypertension, diabetes, benign prostatic hypertrophy, and diverticulosis. Rick does not smoke or use alcohol.

Answers to this chapter begin on page 197.

Exercise 5-49: *Fill-in*
Briefly explain the pathophysiology underlying Parkinson's disease:

_____

_____

_____

Exercise 5-50: *Multiple-choice question*
The imbalance of excitatory and inhibitory neurotransmitters that occurs in Parkinson's disease results in impairment of the:

      A. Extrapyramidal tracts that control semiautomatic function and coordinated movements
      B. Pyramidal tracts, which lead to loss of voluntary movement
      C. Motor cortex, which leads to difficulty with ambulation
      D. Pyramidal tracts and motor cortex, leading to problems with balance

ⓔ   **eResource 5-35:** To reinforce your understanding of the pathophysiology of Parkinson's disease, consult Medscape: [Pathway: Medscape → enter "parkinson" into the search field → select "Parkinson Disease" → review "pathophysiology" under the "Overview" tab]

The nurse asks Rick how he has been and what symptoms he has been experiencing. Rick's wife reports that she can see his symptoms progressing over time. She verbalizes that she is scared of him falling and hurting himself.

Exercise 5-51: *Fill-in*
Identify the four cardinal signs used to diagnose Parkinson's disease:

   1. _____

   2. _____

   3. _____

   4. _____

Exercise 5-52: *Fill-in*
Describe how the following signs manifest in a patient with Parkinson's disease:

   1. Tremors _____

   2. Rigidity _____

   3. Bradykinesia _____

   4. Postural instability _____

ⓔ   **eResource 5-36:** To learn more about the manifestations of Parkinson's disease, view *An Introduction to Parkinson's Disease* by Brian Magennis: http://youtu.be/YVEv9ulfqd4

Answers to this chapter begin on page 197.

Exercise 5-53: *Select all that apply*

Identify other clinical manifestations associated with Parkinson's disease:

- ❏ Excessive, uncontrolled sweating
- ❏ Dementia
- ❏ Decline in intellect
- ❏ Micrographia
- ❏ Masklike, expressionless faces
- ❏ Aphasia
- ❏ Dysphonia

eResource 5-37: To reinforce your understanding of the clinical presentation of Parkinson's disease, review

- ■ Online: Merck Manual: [Pathway: www.merckmanuals.com → select "Merck Manual of Diagnosis and Therapy" → enter "Parkinson" into search field → select "parkinson's disease" → select "Symptoms and Signs" to view content]
- ■ On your mobile device, Medscape: [Pathway: Medscape → enter "parkinson" into the search field → select "parkinson's disease" → select "clinical presentation" and review content]

The PCP is in to see Rick; he asks Rick's wife if she has noticed any new symptoms and how he is tolerating his medications. She reports that she has not noticed anything new, just a gradual overall decline. She asks if there is anything else that can be done.

Exercise 5-54: *Fill-in*

Identify the most effective drug for treating Parkinson's disease and briefly describe its action:

_____

_____

Exercise 5-55: *Select all that apply*

Identify clinical manifestations of dyskinesia that can occur with prolonged use of levodopa:

- ❏ Hallucinations
- ❏ Facial grimaces
- ❏ Sleep alteration
- ❏ Rhythmic jerking of hands
- ❏ Chewing, smacking movements
- ❏ Involuntary movements of the trunk and extremities

eResource 5-38: To better understand dyskinesia and how it is manifested in patients, view the following videos:
- *Parkinson's Disease Symptoms #3: Dyskinesia:*
  http://youtu.be/GgvswR95WQc
- *What Are the Symptoms of Parkinson's Disease?—Ask the Experts:*
  http://youtu.be/IHDFQfmkKlg

Exercise 5-56: *Matching*

Match the drug used to treat Parkinson's disease in Column A with its drug classification in Column B.

Column A	Column B
A. benztropine mesylate (Cogentin)	_____ Catechol-o-methyltransferase inhibitor
B. rasagiline (Azilect)	_____ Anticholinergic agent
C. ropinirole HCl (Requip)	_____ Monoamine oxidase inhibitor
D. entacapone (Comtan)	_____ Dopamine agonist

Exercise 5-57: *Multiple-choice question*

When the wife asks if surgery is an option for treating Parkinson's disease, the best response is:

A. "Surgery costs a lot of money that your insurance probably won't pay for."

B. "Surgery may provide symptom relief, but it does not change the course of the disease or produce permanent improvement."

C. "Surgery is usually reserved for younger people with a longer life expectancy."

D. "Surgery will likely not be successful since he has had Parkinson's disease for 3 years."

 eResource 5-39: To supplement patient teaching, the nurse provides the following information to Rick and his wife:
- Online: Merck Manual: [Pathway: www.merckmanuals.com → select "Merck Manual of Diagnosis and Therapy" → enter "parkinson" into the search field → select "Treatment" and review content]
- Epocrates Online: [Pathway: http//:online.epocrates.com → select "Merck Manual of Diagnosis and Therapy" → enter "parkinson" into the search field → select "follow-up" and review content]
- On your mobile device, Medscape: [Pathway: Medscape → enter "parkinson" into the search field → select "parkinson's disease" → select "Treatment and Management" and review content]

The nurse uses this appointment as an opportunity to discuss interventions that can help Rick and his wife manage his Parkinson's disease. She asks them to identify any difficulties in the home environment so that she can talk to them about possible solutions.

Answers to this chapter begin on page 197.

Exercise 5-58: *Fill-in*

Identify three potential nursing diagnoses for the patient diagnosed with Parkinson's disease:

1. _____

2. _____

3. _____

 eResource 5-40: For more information to help in the development of a nursing care plan for Rick, refer to NANDA Nursing Blogspot: http://goo.gl/1SGo7

Exercise 5-59: *True or false*

Identify whether the following nursing interventions for the patient with Parkinson's disease are true or false:

_____ 1. Warm baths and exercise are recommended to relax muscles and relieve muscle spasms.

_____ 2. Patients should be taught to lean forward when walking to assist with balance.

_____ 3. Walking, swimming, and riding a stationary bicycle help maintain joint mobility.

_____ 4. Patients should be encouraged to remain independent and avoid the use of assistive devices.

Exercise 5-60: *Multiple-choice question*

After educating Rick and his wife about preventing constipation, the nurse determines that the wife understands the information when she states:

A. "He should be taking a daily laxative like Metamucil."

B. "He should be sitting down and attempting to move his bowels at least three times a day."

C. "He needs to increase his fluid intake and eat more foods with fiber."

D. "He needs to drink at least 2 cups of prune juice per day."

 eResource 5-41: For more information regarding strategies to prevent constipation, review information provided in:
■ Medscape: [Pathway: Medscape → enter "constipation" into the search field → select "constipation" → review content under "Treatment and Management"]
■ Careplans Online: http://goo.gl/WFZr7

Exercise 5-61: *Multiple-choice question*

What diet is recommended for patients with Parkinson's disease who are having difficulties with swallowing and choking?

A. Semisolid foods with thin liquids

B. Pureed foods with thin liquids

Answers to this chapter begin on page 197.

C. Solid foods with thick liquids

D. Semisolid foods with thick liquids

Rick and his wife leave his appointment with new information on managing his Parkinson's disease at home. He will continue to be followed closely by his PCP.

 eResource 5-42: For more information regarding long-term monitoring for Rick, refer to:
■ Medscape: [Pathway: Medscape → Parkinson's Disease → "Treatment and Management" → select "long-term monitoring" and review content]
■ Epocrates Online: [Pathway: http://online.epocrates.com → enter "parkinson" into the search field → select "follow-up" and review content]

Unfolding Case Study #35 ▬ Harry

Harry is a 77-year-old male who is seeing his primary care provider (PCP) at the urging of his wife, who has noticed increasing forgetfulness on his part. Although Harry has been forgetful for a few years now, it is starting to become more evident to his family and friends. The PCP completes a health history and physical examination. He orders the following laboratory tests and radiographic exams:

- Complete blood count (CBC)
- Complete metabolic panel (CMP)
- Vitamin B$_{12}$ level
- Thyroid function tests
- Magnetic resonance imaging (MRI)
- Electroencephalography (EEG)

Harry is instructed to make a follow-up appointment when all tests are completed.

Exercise 5-62: *Multiple-choice question*
Alzheimer's disease is most reliably diagnosed by:

A. Excluding all known causes of other dementias or reversible confusion

B. Screening for depression and mental illness

C. MRI or CT scan

D. Examination of cerebrospinal fluid

Exercise 5-63: *Fill-in*

_____ can mimic early-stage Alzheimer's disease, so it is important to rule this out as a problem.

eResource 5-43: To learn more about key findings associated with Alzheimer's disease, consult Epocrates Online: [Pathway: http//:online .epocrates.com → enter "Alzheimer" into search field → select "Alzheimer's disease" and review key findings]

When Harry and his wife return for his follow-up appointment, they are anxious for his results. The PCP informs them that the tests are essentially normal, which leads him to the diagnosis of early Alzheimer's disease. Harry admits that he has been most afraid of this happening. The provider spends extra time with Harry and his wife answering questions.

 eResource 5-44: For more information to supplement patient and family teaching, refer to:
■ National Institutes of Health's (NIH's) *About Alzheimer's Disease: Alzheimer's Basics*: http://goo.gl/E496x
■ NIH Senior Health, *Alzheimer's Disease*: http://goo.gl/KfJ9b
■ National Institute on Aging's publication, *Understanding Alzheimer's Disease: What You Need to Know*: http://goo.gl/RgDPo

Exercise 5-64: *Fill-in*
Briefly describe the pathophysiology of Alzheimer's disease:

_____

_____

Exercise 5-65: *Select all that apply*
Identify clinical manifestations associated with Alzheimer's disease:
❑ Inability to remember familiar faces, places, or objects
❑ Difficulty finding the correct words
❑ Speaking skills deteriorate
❑ Ataxia
❑ Inability to recognize consequences
❑ Difficulty with everyday activities
❑ Personality changes
❑ Hemiparesis

 eResource 5-45: To reinforce your understanding about Alzheimer's disease, view this brief video, *What Is Alzheimer's Disease?*: http://youtu.be/9Wv9jrk-gXc

The provider orders the following medications for Harry:
■ donepezil hydrochloride (Aricept) 5 mg orally daily
■ memantine (Namenda) 5 mg orally daily
Harry is informed that both of these medication dosages can be gradually increased if his symptoms warrant.

Answers to this chapter begin on page 197.

Exercise 5-66: *Fill-in*

Briefly describe the action of donepezil hydrochloride (Aricept):

_____

_____

eResource 5-46: To reinforce your understanding of Aricept, refer to your mobile device and open:
- Epocrates: [Pathway: Epocrates → enter "Aricept" into the search field → review content]
- Medscape: [Pathway: Medscape → enter "Aricept" into the search field → review content]

Exercise 5-67: *Fill-in*

The primary goal in treating Alzheimer's disease is to manage _____ and _____ symptoms.

When the provider is done talking with Harry and his wife, the nurse comes in to review some nursing interventions that will be helpful for care of Harry in the home environment. The goal is to promote independence for as long as possible.

Exercise 5-68: *True or false*

Identify whether the following nursing interventions for the patient with Alzheimer's disease are true or false:

_____ 1. Encourage large family visits to avoid isolation

_____ 2. Organize daily activities into short achievable steps to promote a sense of accomplishment

_____ 3. Keep the environment familiar and noise-free to avoid overreaction to excessive stimulation

_____ 4. Encourage frequent, long naps throughout the day for adequate rest

Exercise 5-69: *Select all that apply*

Identify nursing interventions that support cognitive functioning:

❏ Establish a regular routine

❏ Tell people when they are repeating the same story

❏ Provide simple explanations

❏ Constantly reorient to reality

❏ Use memory aids and cues

❏ Prominently display clocks and calendars

Answers to this chapter begin on page 197.

Exercise 5-70: *Multiple-choice question*

After talking to Harry and his wife about safety measures, the nurse determines that the wife needs further education when she states:

    A. "All potential hazards should be removed from the living areas."

    B. "It is important to keep the house adequately lighted, especially the stairs and bathroom."

    C. "He will be able to continue managing our financial affairs."

    D. "Handrails in the shower and beside the commode may be useful in the future."

 eResource 5-47: For more information about safety precautions, read *Staying Safe*: http://goo.gl/fvObe

Exercise 5-71: *Multiple-choice question*

Patients with Alzheimer's disease prefer foods that are:

    A. Cold and soft

    B. Hot and spicy

    C. New and interesting

    D. Familiar and taste good

Harry's wife begins crying. She states that this is so overwhelming for them.

Exercise 5-72: *Multiple-choice question*

When Harry's wife is distressed and expresses her fears, the nurse's best response is:

    A. "I know how you must feel; this is a terrible diagnosis."

    B. "This must be overwhelming; there are support groups available to help."

    C. "This is hard now, but it will get better."

    D. "You shouldn't cry in front of your husband like this."

When Harry and his wife leave the provider's office, they are planning on talking to their family tonight. They are also going to investigate support groups and various community resources. Both are scared of what the future holds, but they are determined to face it together.

 eResource 5-48: For more information to help Harry's wife locate more resources to support caregiving, refer to:

    ▨ Strategies for Caring for Someone With Alzheimer's: http://goo.gl/u7ZZh

    ▨ Short video describing strategies for managing activities for patients with Alzheimer's: http://goo.gl/ddfm9

Answers to this chapter begin on page 197.

Answers

Exercise 5-1: *Fill-in*

Since the cause of Austin's seizures is unknown, he would be classified as having **primary (idiopathic)** epilepsy.

Exercise 5-2: *Select all that apply*

Identify other potential causes of seizures:

☐ Diabetes—NO

☒ **Head injuries—YES**

☒ **Fever—YES**

☐ Lung cancer—NO

☒ **Brain tumors—YES**

☒ **Central nervous system infections—YES**

☐ Excessive smoking—NO

Exercise 5-3: *Fill-in*

Based upon the information provided by Austin's friends, this would be classified as a **generalized** seizure.

Exercise 5-4: *Fill-in*

Briefly explain the pathophysiology underlying seizures:

An electrical disturbance occurs in an area of nerve cells resulting in abnormal, recurring, uncontrolled electrical discharges. Parts of the body controlled by these nerve cells begin performing erratically.

Exercise 5-5: *Select all that apply*

Identify clinical manifestations associated with generalized seizures:

☒ **Epileptic cry—YES, results from simultaneous contraction of the diaphragm and chest muscles.**

☒ **Tonic-clonic contraction—YES, alternating relaxation and contraction.**

☐ Unintelligible speech—NO, this occurs in simple partial seizures.

☐ Excessive emotions—NO, this occurs in complex partial seizures.

☒ **Incontinence of urine or stool—YES**

☒ **Tongue biting—YES**

Exercise 5-6: *Fill-in*

An aura is a **visual, auditory**, or **olfactory** premonitory or warning sensation.

Exercise 5-7: *Select all that apply*

Identify the most common side effects associated with chronic phenytoin (Dilantin) use:

❑ Aplastic anemia—NO

☒ **Gingival hyperplasia—YES, this is swollen, tender gums.**

☒ **Nausea—YES**

☒ **Nystagmus—YES, this is involuntary back and forth or cyclical movement of the eyes.**

❑ Agranulocytosis—NO

☒ **Hirsutism—YES, this is excessive hair growth or the presence of hair in unusual places.**

Exercise 5-8: *Matching*

Match the generic anticonvulsant medication in Column A with its trade name in Column B.

Column A	Column B	
A. carbamazepine	**D**	Keppra
B. clonazepam	**C**	Neurontin
C. gabapentin	**A**	Tegretol
D. levetiracetam	**E**	Depakote
E. valproate	**B**	Klonopin

Exercise 5-9: *Fill-in*

Identify three potential nursing diagnoses relevant to the patient with a history of seizures:

1. **Risk for injury related to seizure activity**
2. **Fear related to possibility of seizures occurring**
3. **Deficient knowledge related to seizures and their control**

Exercise 5-10: *True or false*

Identify whether the following interventions for epilepsy are true or false:

__True__ 1. Adhering to the prescribed medication regimen, with periodic monitoring of drug levels, is essential for controlling seizures.

__True__ 2. Alcoholic beverages should be avoided because they can increase the risk of seizures.

__False__ 3. At home, patients with epilepsy are advised to purchase padded side rails for their beds.

__True__ 4. Patients are advised to avoid sleep deprivation, which may lower the seizure threshold.

Exercise 5-11: *Multiple-choice question*

A ketogenic diet, which has been found effective in controlling seizures in children, consists of:

A. High-protein, high-carbohydrate, low-fat foods—NO, high carbs are not recommended.

B. Low-protein, high-carbohydrate, low-fat foods—NO, high carbs are not recommended.

C. Low-protein, low-carbohydrate, high-fat foods—NO, high protein is needed.

D. High-protein, low-carbohydrate, high-fat foods—YES

Exercise 5-12: *Multiple-choice question*

When Austin's mother asks if there are any other factors that may precipitate a seizure, the nurse's best response is:

A. "He just needs to take his medication like it is ordered."—NO, the mother is requesting more information.

B. "Emotional states, environmental stressors, or fever can trigger a seizure." YES, try to minimize anxiety and frustration.

C. "The start of menstruation can cause a seizure to occur."—NO, this is not relevant since Austin is male.

D. "He should stop playing video games and watching television because they can precipitate seizures."—NO, photic stimulation (bright flickering lights) can precipitate seizures, but dark glasses or covering one eye may be preventive; it is not realistic to think he will completely stop these activities.

Exercise 5-13: *Select all that apply*

Identify safety-related interventions relevant for the patient with epilepsy:

☒ **Educate family and close friends about patient care during a seizure—YES**

❑ Notify all patient contacts about the patient's diagnosis of epilepsy—NO, only those close to the patient need to be informed and educated.

☒ **Inform all health care providers of medications being taken—YES, many drug interactions can occur with anticonvulsants.**

☒ **Encourage patients to wear a medical information bracelet—YES**

Exercise 5-14: *Multiple-choice question*

After educating Austin's friends about care during a seizure, the nurse determines that they understand the information when one of them states:

A. "We should protect his head, but not attempt to restrain him."—YES, restraining the patient could result in injury.

B. "We should try to open his mouth so he doesn't bite his tongue."—NO, this could cause further injury to the teeth, lips, and tongue.

C. "We should try to get him in the car to bring him to the hospital."—NO, do not attempt to move the person when seizing.

D. "We should keep him on his back after the seizure until help arrives."—NO, if possible, place the person on his or her side with the head flexed forward to keep the tongue forward and to facilitate drainage of saliva.

Exercise 5-15: *Select all that apply*
Identify the risk factors for ischemic stroke that are modifiable:

☐ Age—NO

☒ **Hypertension—YES, this is a major risk factor and control is the key to preventing stroke.**

☒ **Atrial fibrillation—YES, this causes cardiogenic embolic strokes.**

☒ **Hyperlipidemia—YES**

☐ Race—NO

☒ **Smoking—YES**

Exercise 5-16: *Fill-in*
Briefly explain the pathophysiology underlying ischemic strokes:
Cerebral blood flow is interrupted from obstruction of a blood vessel. This initiates the ischemic cascade. A loss of function results if timely intervention does not occur.

Exercise 5-17: *Fill-in*
An ischemic area of brain tissue surrounding the infarcted area, the **penumbra region**, can be salvaged with timely intervention.

Exercise 5-18: *Select all that apply*
Identify clinical manifestations associated with ischemic strokes:

☒ **Hemiplegia or hemiparesis—YES, this is paralysis or weakness on one side of the body.**

☒ **Confusion or change in mental status—YES**

☐ Shortness of breath—NO

☒ **Dysphasia or aphasia—YES, this is impaired or loss of speech.**

☐ Blindness—NO, patients may lose half of their visual field.

☒ **Sensory loss—YES, agnosia is the inability to recognize previously familiar objects.**

☒ **Psychological effects—YES, depression, emotional lability, and frustration may occur.**

Exercise 5-19: *Matching*
Match the stroke location in Column A with its common symptoms/behaviors in Column B. Answers in Column A can be used more than once.

Column A	Column B
A. Right hemispheric stroke	__A__ Paralysis on left side of body
B. Left hemispheric stroke	__B__ Aphasia
	__B__ Slow, cautious behavior
	__A__ Spatial-perceptual deficits
	__B__ Altered intellectual ability
	__A__ Impulsive behavior and poor judgment

Exercise 5-20: *Fill-in*

Identify five contraindications to administering thrombolytic therapy:

1. **Less than 18 years of age**
2. **Onset of stroke symptoms greater than 3 hours**
3. **Systolic blood pressure more than 185 mm Hg and diastolic more than 110 mm Hg**
4. **Currently taking warfarin (Coumadin)**
5. **Platelet count less than 100,000/mm³**
6. **History of intracranial hemorrhage or aneurysm**
7. **Major surgery in the past 2 weeks**
8. **Gastrointestinal or urinary bleeding in the past 3 weeks**

Exercise 5-21: *Calculation*

Order: t-PA dose is 0.9 mg/kg with a maximum dose of 90 mg. Ten percent is to be given IV bolus over 1 minute. The remaining 90% is to be given over 1 hour via infusion pump.

Calculate the total dose of t-PA: **90 mg**

Calculate the amount to be administered over 1 minute: **9 mg**

Calculate the amount to be administered over 1 hour: **81 mg**

Exercise 5-22: *Select all that apply*

Identify factors associated with the occurrence of intracranial bleeding post t-PA:

☒ **Age greater than 70 years—YES**

☒ **Serum glucose 300 mg/dL or greater—YES**

❑ Increased calcium levels—NO

☒ **Cerebral edema on patient's first CT scan—YES**

❑ African American race—NO

❑ Male gender—NO

Exercise 5-23: *Fill-in*

Identify three potential nursing diagnoses for the patient diagnosed with an ischemic stroke:

1. **Impaired physical mobility related to hemiparesis, loss of balance, and brain injury**
2. **Self-care deficit (bathing, toileting, grooming, feeding) related to brain injury**
3. **Impaired swallowing related to brain injury**
4. **Impaired verbal communication related to brain injury**
5. **Interrupted family processes related to illness and caregiver burden**

Exercise 5-24: *True or false*

Identify whether the following nursing interventions for care of the stroke patient are true or false:

False 1. Unaffected extremities are exercised passively three to four times a day to maintain joint mobility and regain motor control.

True 2. Patients are first taught to maintain sitting and standing balance before attempting ambulation.

True 3. Instruct patients to carry out self-care activities on the unaffected side.

False 4. Health care personnel should assist patients with expressive aphasia by finishing their thoughts or sentences.

Exercise 5-25: *Multiple-choice question*

When Pam's daughter asks why her mother is not receiving as much help as when she was in the hospital, the nurse's best response is:

A. "We have fewer nurses and patient care technicians than the hospitals."—NO

B. "She needs to learn to take care of herself now."—NO

C. "Usually the families help with the patient's care."—NO

D. **"We are trying to help your mother regain as much independence as possible."—YES, this helps to explain why the patient is being encouraged to do more for herself.**

Exercise 5-26: *Fill-in*

Identify five assistive devices designed to improve the self-care of stroke patients:

1. **Wide-grip utensils to help with weak grasps**
2. **Shower and tub seats**
3. **Raised toilet seats**
4. **Velcro closures**
5. **Canes, walkers, or wheelchairs**
6. **Plate guards to prevent food from being pushed off**
7. **Long-handled bath sponge**
8. **Grab bars next to toilet**
9. **Elastic shoelaces**

Exercise 5-27: *Multiple-choice question*

After talking to Pam's husband and daughter about the potential effects of caregiving on the family, the nurse determines that the daughter understands the information when she states:

A. "Dad needs to take on all of Mom's responsibilities now."—NO, Pam needs to be encouraged to continue those responsibilities of which she is capable; her husband cannot be expected to take on all responsibilities.

B. "Dad needs to remain close to Mom at all times while at home."—NO, Pam needs supervision, but she doesn't need to be in constant sight.

C. **"Mom is going to initially need 24-hour supervision, so we need to plan ways to give Dad a break."—YES, this is important in preventing caregiver strain and depression.**

D. "Dad has always looked out for Mom, so he will have no trouble taking her home."—NO, some adaptation will be required.

Exercise 5-28: *Select all that apply*

Identify risk factors for spinal cord injuries:

☒ **Young age—YES, 50% of injured are 16 to 30 years of age.**

☒ **Alcohol use—YES**

☐ Smoking—NO

☐ African American race—NO, 62% of injured are Caucasian.

☒ **Drug use—YES**

☒ **Male gender—YES**

Exercise 5-29: *Ordering*

Rank the causes of spinal cord injuries in order of their frequency of occurrence:

___4___ Recreational sporting activities

___2___ Falls

___3___ Violence (gunshot wounds)

___1___ Motor vehicle accidents

Exercise 5-30: *Multiple-choice question*

In order to prevent further damage when moving a patient with a potential spinal cord injury, it is important to:

A. Place the patient in a side-lying position for transport.—NO, the patient should be supine on the backboard.

B. Place the patient in traction shortly after arrival in the emergency department.—NO, the need for traction depends on the injury and is ordered by the neurosurgeon.

C. Avoid all radiographic exams until the injury has been ruled out by neurological examination.—NO, these exams are necessary to aid in diagnosis.

D. **Keep the patient immobilized on a backboard with the head and neck maintained in a neutral position.—YES, limit the patient's head movement to prevent flexion, rotation, and extension.**

Exercise 5-31: *Calculation*

Order: methylprednisolone 30 mg/kg IV over 15 minutes

   Patient's weight is 198 pounds

Calculate the dose of methylprednisolone: **2700 mg**

Exercise 5-32: *Select all that apply*

Identify acute complications that can occur after a spinal cord injury:

- ❑ Myocardial infarction—NO, patients with spinal cord injury are generally young with no heart disease.
- ☒ **Neurogenic shock—YES, this is related to a loss of autonomic nervous system function below the level of the injury.**
- ☒ **Deep vein thrombosis—YES, related to immobility.**
- ☒ **Respiratory complications—YES, pneumonia and respiratory failure may occur.**
- ❑ Stroke—NO
- ☒ **Autonomic dysreflexia—YES**

Exercise 5-33: *Fill-in*

Identify five potential nursing diagnoses for the patient diagnosed with acute spinal cord injury:

1. **Ineffective breathing pattern related to weakness of abdominal and intercostal muscles**
2. **Ineffective airway clearance related to weakness of intercostal muscles**
3. **Impaired physical mobility related to motor impairment**
4. **Disturbed sensory perception related to sensory impairment**
5. **Impaired urinary elimination related to disruption of reflexes**
6. **Risk for impaired skin integrity related to immobility**

Exercise 5-34: *True or false*

Identify whether the following nursing interventions for the patient with a spinal cord injury are true or false:

__True__ 1. Breathing exercises are encouraged for strengthening of inspiratory muscles.

__False__ 2. Passive range-of-motion is discouraged below the level of spinal cord injury.

__False__ 3. Vigorous suctioning should be used frequently to prevent retention of secretions.

__True__ 4. Splints, which are used to prevent footdrop, should be removed and reapplied every 2 hours.

Exercise 5-35: *Multiple-choice question*

When Dean's mother asks what can be done to keep his skin in good condition, the nurse's best response is:

A. "Unfortunately, it is inevitable that he will develop skin breakdown at some point."—NO, this is not necessarily true and certainly not helpful.

B. "Most importantly, we need to turn and reposition him at least every 2 hours." YES, this prevents pressure ulcers, pooling of blood, and edema in dependent areas.

C. "Using lotion once a day will keep his skin smooth and soft."—NO, this is not the primary method of preventing skin breakdown.

D. "They will teach you that information before he leaves the rehabilitation facility."—NO, the family should be involved in the patient's care from the very beginning.

Exercise 5-36: *Multiple-choice question*

Patients are initially allowed nothing by mouth (NPO) after a spinal cord injury, but once bowel sounds return, they should begin a diet that is:

A. High-calorie, high-protein, high-fiber—YES, the high-calorie and high-protein are important for healing; the high-fiber is important in preventing constipation.

B. Low-calorie, high-protein, low-fiber—NO, fiber is needed due to immobility.

C. Low-calorie, high-protein, high-fiber—NO, calories are needed for healing.

D. High-calorie, high-protein, low-fiber—NO, fiber is needed due to immobility.

Exercise 5-37: *Select all that apply*

Identify interventions designed to minimize the risk of thrombophlebitis in the patient with an acute spinal cord injury:

☒ **Anticoagulation—YES, heparin subcutaneously or warfarin (Coumadin) orally may be used.**

☐ Abdominal binders—NO, this may assist venous return, but will not help in the extremities, where there is greatest risk.

☒ **Antiembolism stockings—YES, promotes venous return.**

☒ **Adequate hydration—YES**

☐ Antiplatelet medications—NO, this is not helpful in preventing venous thrombi.

☒ **Pneumatic compression devices—YES, decreases venous pooling and promotes venous return.**

Exercise 5-38: *Multiple-choice question*

When Dean is heard telling a friend that he will never be anything but a burden for his family, the nurse's best response is:

A. "Your family loves you and will take good care of you."—NO, this does not increase independence.

B. "You should be thinking more positive thoughts."—NO, this minimizes the patient's feelings.

C. **"In rehabilitation, they will be teaching you how to care for yourself."—YES, many patients can achieve self-care and some degree of independence.**

D. "Unfortunately, you will always have to live with your family."—NO, this is not true.

Exercise 5-39: *Fill-in*
Briefly explain the pathophysiology underlying multiple sclerosis:
A damaged immune system causes inflammation, which in turn destroys the myelin sheath throughout the central nervous system. Demyelination interrupts the flow of nerve impulses.

Exercise 5-40: *Select all that apply*
Identify other clinical manifestations associated with multiple sclerosis:

☒ **Depression—YES**

☒ **Numbness—YES**

☐ Dizziness—NO

☒ **Visual disturbances—YES, blurred vision, diplopia, or blindness may occur.**

☒ **Loss of balance—YES**

☒ **Pain—YES, occurs with lesions on sensory pathways.**

☐ Diarrhea—NO

☒ **Cognitive changes—YES, memory loss or decreased concentration may occur.**

Exercise 5-41: *Multiple-choice question*
On MRI, patients with multiple sclerosis have:
A. Increased cerebral spinal fluid—NO
B. Atrophy of gray matter—NO
C. **Multiple plaques throughout the central nervous system—YES**
D. Inflammation of the basal ganglia—NO

Exercise 5-42: *Fill-in*
Identify five potential side effects that may occur with administration of glatiramer (Copaxone):

1. **Flu-like symptoms**
2. **Anxiety**
3. **Weakness**
4. **Rashes**
5. **Nausea**
6. **Diarrhea**
7. **Urgency**
8. **Injection site reactions**

Exercise 5-43: *Ordering*
Number in order the steps required for administration of glatiramer (Copaxone):
- **3** Choose injection site in arms, thigh, or abdomen
- **6** Discard needle in puncture-resistant container
- **1** Allow prefilled syringe to warm to room temperature for 20 minutes
- **5** Pinch skin and inject at a 90-degree angle
- **2** Inspect medication to ensure it is clear and colorless to slightly yellow
- **4** Clean site with alcohol and allow to dry

Exercise 5-44: *True or false*
Identify whether the following strategies for controlling fatigue associated with multiple sclerosis are true or false:
- **False** 1. Avoid cold environments and temperatures
- **True** 2. Achieve a balance between rest and activities
- **False** 3. Stop all medications when fatigue becomes severe
- **True** 4. Maintain a healthy lifestyle, avoiding alcohol and smoking

Exercise 5-45: *Fill-in*
Identify three potential nursing diagnoses for the patient diagnosed with multiple sclerosis:
1. **Impaired physical mobility related to weakness and spasticity**
2. **Disturbed thought processes related to changes in the central nervous system**
3. **Ineffective individual coping related to uncertainty of disease process**
4. **Impaired urinary elimination related to central nervous system dysfunction**
5. **Risk for injury related to motor and sensory impairment**

Exercise 5-46: *Select all that apply*
Identify interventions designed to promote physical mobility in the patient with multiple sclerosis:
- ☐ Strenuous activity to the point of fatigue—NO, this can raise body temperature and aggravate symptoms.
- ☒ **Frequent, short rest periods—YES**
- ☒ **Daily exercises for muscle stretching—YES, this prevents joint contractures.**
- ☐ Exercise in a warm environment—NO, this can raise body temperature and aggravate symptoms.
- ☒ **Walking—YES, this helps to improve gait.**
- ☐ Hot baths with spasms—NO, this can raise body temperature and aggravate symptoms; warm packs may be used.

Exercise 5-47: *Multiple-choice question*

If difficulty in coordination occurs as a result of motor dysfunction, it is first recommended to:

A. Watch the feet while walking—NO, this may be helpful if a loss of position sense occurs.

B. Use an assistive device, such as braces—NO, this is not necessary yet.

C. Use a wheelchair or motorized scooter—NO, this is not necessary.

D. Walk with feet apart to widen the base of support—YES, this increases walking stability.

Exercise 5-48: *Multiple-choice question*

When Kacey's mother asks what she can do about Kacey's moodiness, the nurse's best response is:

A. "You need to set limits on her behavior."—NO, this does not support the patient's crises.

B. "Just ignore her and she will quit acting out so much."—NO, this is also unsupportive.

C. "Suggest that she stay in her room until she is in a better mood."—NO, unsupportive.

D. "People adapt to illness differently; support of family and friends is of primary importance."—YES, emotional lability may be a manifestation of her multiple sclerosis.

Exercise 5-49: *Fill-in*

Briefly explain the pathophysiology underlying Parkinson's disease:

Cells in the substantia nigra in the basal ganglia area of the brain are destroyed for unknown reasons resulting in decreased levels of dopamine. The effect of less dopamine results in more excitatory neurotransmitters (acetylcholine) than inhibitory (dopamine).

Exercise 5-50: *Multiple-choice question*

The imbalance of excitatory and inhibitory neurotransmitters that occurs in Parkinson's disease results in impairment of the:

A. Extrapyramidal tracts that control semiautomatic function and coordinated movements—YES, complex body movements are affected.

B. Pyramidal tracts, which lead to loss of voluntary movement—NO, pyramidal tracts are not affected.

C. Motor cortex, which leads to difficulty with ambulation—NO, the motor cortex is not affected.

D. Pyramidal tracts and motor cortex, leading to problems with balance—NO, pyramidal tracts and the motor cortex are not affected.

Exercise 5-51: *Fill-in*

Identify the four cardinal signs used to diagnose Parkinson's disease:

1. **Tremor**
2. **Rigidity**
3. **Bradykinesia**
4. **Postural instability**

Exercise 5-52: *Fill-in*

Describe how the following signs manifest in a patient with Parkinson's disease:

1. Tremor **Occurs at rest; disappears with purposeful movement. May also manifest as pronation-supination of the forearm or "pill rolling."**
2. Rigidity **Stiffness of the arms, legs, face, and posture. Passive movement of an extremity may lead to jerky movements described as a "cog-wheel" movement.**
3. Bradykinesia **Slower movements and difficulty initiating movement.**
4. Postural instability **Loss of postural reflexes occur. Patient walks with head bent and has a propulsive, shuffling gait.**

Exercise 5-53: *Select all that apply*

Identify other clinical manifestations associated with Parkinson's disease:

☒ **Excessive, uncontrolled sweating—YES, this is an autonomic symptom.**

☒ **Dementia—YES, a progressive mental deterioration occurs in about 75% of patients.**

❑ Decline in intellect—NO

☒ **Micrographia—YES, small handwriting develops as dexterity declines.**

☒ **Masklike, expressionless faces—YES**

❑ Aphasia—NO

☒ **Dysphonia—YES, this is a soft, slurred speech.**

Exercise 5-54: *Fill-in*

Identify the most effective drug for treating Parkinson's disease and briefly describe its action:

Levodopa (Larodopa) is the mainstay of treatment for Parkinson's disease. The drug is converted to dopamine in the basal ganglia, thus providing relief of symptoms.

Exercise 5-55: *Select all that apply*

Identify clinical manifestations of dyskinesia that can occur with prolonged use of levodopa:

❑ Hallucinations—NO

☒ **Facial grimaces—YES**

❑ Sleep alteration—NO

☒ **Rhythmic jerking of hands—YES**

☒ **Chewing, smacking movements—YES**

☒ **Involuntary movements of the trunk and extremities—YES**

Exercise 5-56: *Matching*

Match the drug used to treat Parkinson's disease in Column A with its drug classification in Column B.

Column A	Column B
A. benztropine mesylate (Cogentin)	__D__ Catechol-o-methyltransferase inhibitor
B. rasagiline (Azilect)	__A__ Anticholinergic agent
C. ropinirole HCl (Requip)	__B__ Monoamine oxidase inhibitor
D. entacapone (Comtan)	__C__ Dopamine agonist

Exercise 5-57: *Multiple-choice question*

When the wife asks if surgery is an option for treating Parkinson's disease, the best response is:

A. "Surgery costs a lot of money that your insurance probably won't pay for."—NO

B. "Surgery may provide symptom relief, but it does not change the course of the disease or produce permanent improvement."—YES

C. "Surgery is usually reserved for younger people with a longer life expectancy."—NO

D. "Surgery will likely not be successful since he has had Parkinson's disease for 3 years."—NO

Exercise 5-58: *Fill-in*

Identify three potential nursing diagnoses for the patient diagnosed with Parkinson's disease:

1. **Impaired physical mobility related to muscle rigidity**
2. **Self-care deficit related to tremor and motor dysfunction**
3. **Ineffective coping related to disease progression**
4. **Imbalanced nutrition, less than body requirements, related to tremor and slow eating**
5. **Risk for injury-related to motor dysfunction**

Exercise 5-59: *True or false*

Identify whether the following nursing interventions for the patient with Parkinson's disease are true or false:

__True__ 1. Warm baths and exercise are recommended to relax muscles and relieve muscle spasms.

__False__ 2. Patients should be taught to lean forward when walking to assist with balance.

__True__ 3. Walking, swimming, and riding a stationary bicycle help maintain joint mobility.

__False__ 4. Patients should be encouraged to remain independent and avoid the use of assistive devices.

Exercise 5-60: *Multiple-choice question*

After educating Rick and his wife about preventing constipation, the nurse determines that the wife understands the information when she states:

A. "He should be taking a daily laxative like Metamucil."—NO, chronic laxative use is discouraged.

B. "He should be sitting down and attempting to move his bowels at least three times a day."—NO

C. **"He needs to increase his fluid intake and eat more foods with fiber."—YES, this is the best way of preventing constipation.**

D. "He needs to drink at least 2 cups of prune juice per day."—NO

Exercise 5-61: *Multiple-choice question*

What diet is recommended for patients with Parkinson's disease who are having difficulties with swallowing and choking?

A. Semisolid foods with thin liquids—NO, thin liquids should be avoided.

B. Pureed foods with thin liquids—NO, thin liquids should be avoided.

C. Solid foods with thick liquids—NO, solid foods may be harder to swallow.

D. **Semisolid foods with thick liquids—YES, this is easiest to swallow.**

Exercise 5-62: *Multiple-choice question*

Alzheimer's disease is most reliably diagnosed by:

A. **Excluding all known causes of other dementias or reversible confusion—YES, Alzheimer's disease is a diagnosis of exclusion; a definitive diagnosis can only be made at autopsy.**

B. Screening for depression and mental illness—NO, this is not related.

C. MRI or CT scan—NO, these are not reliable for making a diagnosis of Alzheimer's disease.

D. Examination of cerebrospinal fluid—NO, this is not the cause.

Exercise 5-63: *Fill-in*

<u>**Depression**</u> can mimic early stage Alzheimer's disease, so it is important to rule this out as a problem.

Exercise 5-64: *Fill-in*

Briefly describe the pathophysiology of Alzheimer's disease:

<u>**Tangled masses of nonfunctioning neurons and senile plaques develop in the cerebral cortex. Cells that use acetylcholine, which is needed for memory, are primarily affected.**</u>

Exercise 5-65: *Select all that apply*
Identify clinical manifestations associated with Alzheimer's disease:
☒ **Inability to remember familiar faces, places, or objects—YES**
☒ **Difficulty finding the correct words—YES**
☒ **Speaking skills deteriorate—YES**
❑ Ataxia—NO
☒ **Inability to recognize consequences—YES**
☒ **Difficulty with everyday activities—YES**
☒ **Personality changes—YES**
❑ Hemiparesis—NO

Exercise 5-66: *Fill-in*
Briefly describe the action of donepezil hydrochloride (Aricept):
This cholinesterase inhibitor drug inhibits acetylcholinesterase, which makes more acetylcholine available. This does not cure the disease, but helps maintain memory skills.

Exercise 5-67: *Fill-in*
The primary goal in treating Alzheimer's disease is to manage **cognitive** and **behavioral** symptoms.

Exercise 5-68: *True or false*
Identify whether the following nursing interventions for the patient with Alzheimer's disease are true or false:
  False 1. Encourage large family visits to avoid isolation
  True 2. Organize daily activities into short achievable steps to promote a sense of accomplishment
  True 3. Keep the environment familiar and noise-free to avoid overreaction to excessive stimulation
  False 4. Encourage frequent, long naps throughout the day for adequate rest

Exercise 5-69: *Select all that apply*
Identify nursing interventions that support cognitive functioning:
☒ **Establish a regular routine—YES**
❑ Tell people when they are repeating the same story—NO, this may increase anxiety.
☒ **Provide simple explanations—YES**
❑ Constantly reorient to reality—NO, this may increase anxiety.
☒ **Use memory aids and cues—YES**
☒ **Prominently display clocks and calendars—YES**

Exercise 5-70: *Multiple-choice question*

After talking to Harry and his wife about safety measures, the nurse determines that the wife needs further education when she states:

A. "All potential hazards should be removed from the living areas."—NO

B. "It is important to keep the house adequately lighted, especially the stairs and bathroom."—NO

C. "He will be able to continue managing our financial affairs."—YES, as the patient becomes increasingly forgetful, he will be incapable of making good decisions.

D. "Handrails in the shower and beside the commode may be useful in the future."—NO

Exercise 5-71: *Multiple-choice question*

Patients with Alzheimer's disease prefer foods that are:

A. Cold and soft—NO

B. Hot and spicy—NO

C. New and interesting—NO

D. Familiar and taste good—YES

Exercise 5-72: *Multiple-choice question*

When Harry's wife is distressed and expresses her fears, the nurse's best response is:

A. "I know how you must feel; this is a terrible diagnosis."—NO, you can't know how another person feels.

B. "This is must be overwhelming; there are support groups available to help."— YES, there are many community resources available.

C. "This is hard now, but it will get better."—NO, the patient is only going to get progressively worse.

D. "You shouldn't cry in front of your husband like this."—NO, that does not assist communication.

6

Nursing Care of the Patient With Endocrine Disease

Karen K. Gittings

Unfolding Case Study #36 ▮ Jenny

Jenny is a 56-year-old female who is scheduled for a routine primary care provider's (PCP) visit to follow-up on her hypertension. She reports no significant complaints other than her vision being blurry; she states, "I need to go to the eye doctor to have my eyes checked." At the conclusion of her visit, the PCP orders a basic metabolic panel (BMP) and complete blood count (CBC) to be drawn. Jenny receives a phone call 2 days later from her PCP's office to schedule an appointment for later that day. Jenny is told that her blood sugar is elevated. At her appointment, Jenny and the nurse begin by reviewing Jenny's risk factors for diabetes.

Exercise 6-1: *Select all that apply*
Identify risk factors commonly associated with diabetes mellitus:

- ❑ Obesity
- ❑ Age less than 45 years
- ❑ Caucasian race
- ❑ Family history
- ❑ History of gestational diabetes
- ❑ History of delivering babies over 9 pounds

ⓔ **eResource 6-1:** To review risk factors associated with diabetes, consult Epocrates Online: [Pathway: → http://online.epocrates.com → select the "diseases" tab → enter "Diabetes" into the search field → review content related to "risks"]

Jenny reports that her mother and grandmother were diabetics. She is also over 45 years old and overweight at 5 feet 2 inches and 200 pounds. Jenny still finds it hard to believe that she could be diabetic since she is feeling okay; she asks the nurse to explain to her how diabetes occurs.

Exercise 6-2: *Multiple-choice question*

The nurse educating Jenny on type 2 diabetes determines that she understands the information when she states:

      A. "I am not producing any insulin because of a problem with my immune system."

      B. "I will need to take insulin for the rest of my life."

      C. "I'm not making enough insulin or my body isn't as sensitive to it."

      D. "I won't need to make any dietary changes if I take my medicine."

Exercise 6-3: *Matching*

Match the type of diabetes in Column A with its typical characteristics in Column B. Answers in Column A can be used more than once.

Column A	Column B
A. Type 1 diabetes	_____ Onset is usually under 30 years old
B. Type 2 diabetes	_____ Patient is often thin at time of diagnosis
	_____ Treated with diet, exercise, and oral agents
	_____ Patient is often obese at time of diagnosis
	_____ Antibodies are present in the body
	_____ Patients require insulin for life

   (e)   **eResource 6-2:** To learn more about the pathophysiology of type 2 diabetes, open Medscape on your mobile device: [Pathway: Medscape → enter "Type 2 Diabetes" into the search field → in the "overview" section, select "pathophysiology" and review content]

By the time it is Jenny's turn to see her PCP, she has a beginning understanding about diabetes. Her PCP sits with her and begins by reviewing her laboratory results. Her fasting plasma glucose from her last visit was 236 mg/dL. The PCP lists some typical signs and symptoms of diabetes, and he asks Jenny if she is experiencing any of them.

Exercise 6-4: *Select all that apply*

Identify common clinical manifestations associated with diabetes mellitus:

      ❑ Polyuria

      ❑ Decreased appetite

      ❑ Decreased fluid intake

      ❑ Vision changes

      ❑ Fatigue

   (e)   **eResource 6-3:** For more information regarding clinical manifestations associated with diabetes mellitus, refer to the Merck Manual: [Pathway: www.merckmanuals.com → select "Merck Manual of Diagnosis and

Answers to this chapter begin on page 231.

Therapy" → enter "Diabetes" into the search field → select "Diabetes Mellitus (DM)" → select "Symptoms and Signs" and review content]

Jenny reports that her vision has been blurry, but she thought that she needed new glasses. She also recognizes that she has been drinking and urinating more than usual. Based on her symptoms and elevated fasting plasma glucose, the physician suspects Jenny has type 2 diabetes.

 eResource 6-4: To learn more about the diagnostic work-up for Jenny, refer to Medscape on your mobile device: [Pathway: Medscape → enter "Type 2 Diabetes" into the search field → select "Type 2 Diabetes Mellitus" → select "Workup" and review content]

To further confirm the diagnosis, he orders a random fingerstick blood sugar and Hemoglobin A1C (HgbA1C).

Exercise 6-5: *Short answer*
Briefly explain how a HgbA1C is used to evaluate blood glucose compared to a random blood glucose level.

_____

_____

_____

_____

 eResource 6-5: To learn more about HgbA1C, refer to Medscape on your mobile device: [Pathway: Medscape → enter "A1C" into the search field → select "Hemoglobin A1C testing"and review content]

Jenny's blood results are ready within a short period of time. Her fingerstick blood sugar is 286 and her HgbA1C is 9%. Her physician orders metformin 500 mg orally twice a day, and Jenny is scheduled to meet with a diabetes educator in 2 days.

Exercise 6-6: *Fill-in*
Identify three ways in which metformin acts to maintain normal blood glucose levels:

1. _____

2. _____

3. _____

 eResource 6-6: To review patient teaching regarding metformin with Jenny, refer to Epocrates on your mobile device: [Pathway: Epocrates → enter "metformin" into the search field → select "metformin" → scroll down to review "common reactions" and other relevant content]

Jenny meets with the diabetes educator as scheduled. During her appointment, they discuss many topics including nutrition and exercise. The educator begins by talking about meal planning and caloric needs.

Exercise 6-7: *Fill-in*

For obese patients who are diabetic, the key to treatment is: _____.

Exercise 6-8: *Fill-in*

Identify the food groups that are part of the Exchange List system and give one example of a specific food within each group:

1. _____
2. _____
3. _____
4. _____
5. _____
6. _____
7. _____
8. _____

Exercise 6-9: *True or false*

Identify whether the following statements about nutrition in the diabetic patient are true or false:

_____ 1. Soluble fiber lowers blood glucose levels by slowing the rate of glucose absorption from these foods.

_____ 2. Alcohol used in combination with chlorpropamide (Diabinese) may cause facial flushing, warmth, nausea, and vomiting.

_____ 3. Nutritive sweeteners have no effect on blood glucose levels.

Exercise 6-10: *Multiple-choice question*

The nurse educating Jenny on exercise determines that she needs further instruction when she states:

A. "Exercise will lower my blood glucose level."
B. "I should try to exercise at the same time each day."
C. "Walking is generally a safe form of exercise."
D. "I should exercise more when my glucose levels are more than 250 mg/dL."

 eResource 6-7: To learn more about nutritional management of patients with diabetes, refer to Medscape on your mobile device: [Pathway: Medscape → enter "nutrition" into the search field → select "Nutritional Management of Patients with Diabetes" and review content]

Jenny is given a blood glucose monitor with instructions for self-monitoring of her glucose levels. Once Jenny's blood glucose level is stabilized, she is instructed to test at least two to three times per week.

Answers to this chapter begin on page 231.

Exercise 6-11: *Select all that apply*

Identify other circumstances in which more frequent testing is recommended:

- ❑ Missing a mealtime
- ❑ Symptoms of hypoglycemia
- ❑ Changes in medications
- ❑ During periods of increased stress
- ❑ Times of illness

The diabetes educator explains to Jenny how metformin works to control her blood glucose level. Jenny expresses concern that she may have to use insulin if the metformin is ineffective, but the nurse explains that there are many other oral agents available that can be tried before moving to insulin.

Exercise 6-12: *Matching*

Match the medication in Column A with its drug classification and action in Column B.

Column A	Column B
A. chlorpropamide (Diabinese)	_____ Alpha-glucosidase inhibitor; delays intestinal absorption of complex carbs
B. glipizide (Glucotrol)	_____ First-generation sulfonylurea; stimulates beta cells of the pancreas to secrete insulin
C. metformin (Glucophage)	_____ Nonsulfonylurea insulin secretagogue; stimulates the pancreas to secrete insulin
D. acarbose (Precose)	_____ Second-generation sulfonylurea; stimulates beta cells of the pancreas to secrete insulin
E. nateglinide (Starlix)	_____ Biguanide; inhibits production of glucose by the liver

 eResource 6-8: To learn more about these medications, consult Medscape on your mobile device: [Pathway: Medscape → enter "Type 2 Diabetes" → select "Medication" and review content]

As Jenny's appointment draws to an end, the diabetes educator teaches her about hypoglycemia and long-term complications.

Exercise 6-13: *Multiple-choice question*

The nurse educating Jenny on hypoglycemia determines that she understands the information when she states:

- A. "I won't get hypoglycemic when I am only taking metformin."
- B. "If I feel my blood sugar dropping, I will eat some chocolate candy."
- C. "My family should be educated on how to help me if I become hypoglycemic."
- D. "Hypoglycemia most often occurs 1 hour after meals."

Answers to this chapter begin on page 231.

Exercise 6-14: *Fill-in*

Identify the macrovascular and microvascular complications that can occur with diabetes:

Macrovascular	Microvascular
1. _____	1. _____
2. _____	2. _____
3. _____	

eResource 6-9: To learn more about microvascular and macrovascular complications, refer to Medscape on your mobile device: [Pathway: Medscape → enter "Type 2 Diabetes" → select "Treatment and Management" → select "Approach and Considerations" and scroll down to review content]

Exercise 6-15: *Select all that apply*

Identify foot care techniques recommended for diabetic patients:

❑ Assess feet daily

❑ Lotion the feet, especially between the toes

❑ Use hot water for soaking the feet

❑ Trim toenails straight across

❑ Never walk barefoot

eResource 6-10: To supplement patient teaching regarding diabetes, refer to:
- ▨ MedlinePlus's interactive tutorial, *Diabetes—Introduction:* http://goo.gl/nJn7E
- ▨ National Institutes of Health's (NIH's) pamphlet, *Your Guide to Diabetes: Type 1 and Type 2*: http://goo.gl/bgBNl

eResource 6-11: To learn about the American College of Physicians recommended vaccinations for Jenny to help keep her healthy, download the ACP Immunization Advisor (ACP-IA) "app" onto your mobile device (http://goo.gl/NZQJB). [Pathway on your mobile device: ACP-IA → select "find" → enter "age" and "Condition" (Note: There are no special considerations for Jenny) → select "Show Vaccines"]

Unfolding Case Study #37 ▨ Lorrie

Lorrie is a 60-year-old female who was recently diagnosed with hypothyroidism. Her granddaughter, Alissa, who is in college studying to be a registered nurse, is very interested in learning more about hypothyroidism so that she can help to educate her grandmother about her disease process. Alissa begins by reviewing basic anatomy and physiology of the thyroid gland.

Answers to this chapter begin on page 231.

Exercise 6-16: *Select all that apply*

Identify the hormones released by the thyroid gland:

❑ Thyroxine (T4)

❑ Thyroid-stimulating hormone (TSH)

❑ Triiodothyronine (T3)

❑ Calcitonin

❑ Antidiuretic hormone (ADH)

Exercise 6-17: *Fill-in*

Essential for the synthesis of thyroid hormones, _____ is obtained through diet.

Exercise 6-18: *Short answer*

Briefly explain how the release of thyroid hormone is regulated in the body.

_____

_____

_____

_____

_____

eResource 6-12: To learn more, Alissa refers to Medscape on her mobile device: [Pathway: Medscape → enter "hypothyroidism" → select "Overview" → review content listed under "Background," "Epidemiology," and "Pathophysiology"]

Alissa is aware that many endocrine disorders have general signs and symptoms, which may be initially ignored or thought of as being a part of the normal aging process. Alissa asks her grandmother what types of signs and symptoms she was experiencing.

Exercise 6-19: *Fill-in*

Identify three common signs and symptoms that may indicate an endocrine disorder:

1. _____

2. _____

3. _____

eResource 6-13: To learn more about common signs and symptoms associated with an endocrine disorder, refer to the Merck Manual:

▪ Hypothyroidism: [Pathway: www.merckmanuals.com → select "Merck Manual of Diagnosis and Therapy" → enter "hypothyroidism" into the search field → select "hypothyroidism" → select "Symptoms and Signs" and review content]

▪ Endocrine Disorders: [Pathway: www.merckmanuals.com → select "Merck Manual of Diagnosis and Therapy" → enter "Endocrine Disorders" into the search field → select "Endocrine Disorders" and review content]

Answers to this chapter begin on page 231.

Lorrie tells her granddaughter that she had been feeling very tired and had little energy for cleaning the house or family activities. Because she didn't initially think anything was really wrong, Lorrie did not seek medical attention, but waited until her regularly scheduled primary care provider's (PCP) appointment 3 months later to mention her fatigue. Her PCP ordered some laboratory tests to be done on that day and scheduled her for a follow-up appointment in 1 week.

Exercise 6-20: *Select all that apply*
Identify clinical manifestations associated with hypothyroidism:

❑ Weight loss

❑ Fatigue

❑ Irritability

❑ Hair loss

❑ Increased pulse

❑ Feeling cold in a warm environment

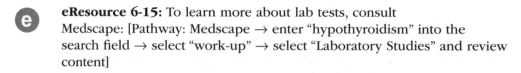 **eResource 6-14:** To learn more about the clinical presentation, refer to Medscape: [Pathway: Medscape → enter "hypothyroidism" into the search field → select "clinical presentation" and review content]

Exercise 6-21: *Matching*
Match the laboratory test in Column A with its description and normal value in Column B.

Column A	Column B
A. TSH	_____ 70% is protein-bound; normal is 5 to 11 mcg/dL
B. T3	_____ Direct measurement of unbound thyroxine; normal is 0.8 to 2.7 ng/dL
C. T4	_____ Best screening test for thyroid function; normal is 0.4 to 4.2 mIU/L
D. Free T4	_____ More accurate indicator of hyperthyroidism; normal is 70 to 204 ng/dL

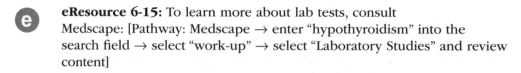 **eResource 6-15:** To learn more about lab tests, consult Medscape: [Pathway: Medscape → enter "hypothyroidism" into the search field → select "work-up" → select "Laboratory Studies" and review content]

At her follow-up appointment, Lorrie received her diagnosis of hypothyroidism and was started on levothyroxine (Synthroid) 0.075 mg orally daily. Later, Alissa reviews the medication with her grandmother so that she clearly understands the need to continue taking it as directed.

Exercise 6-22: *True or false*

Identify whether the following statements about thyroid hormone replacement therapy are true or false:

     _____ 1. TSH levels are used for monitoring the effectiveness of thyroid hormone replacement and in making dosage adjustments of the medications.

     _____ 2. Signs of overdose are manifested as hyperthyroidism (tachycardia, weight loss, nervousness, and/or chest pain).

     _____ 3. Thyroid hormone replacement is only needed until symptoms subside; the medication can then be discontinued.

 eResource 6-16: To learn more about this medication, Alissa consults Epocrates on her mobile device: [Pathway: Epocrates → enter "Synthroid" into the search field → review content]

Since Lorrie has only recently been diagnosed with hypothyroidism and started on levothyroxine (Synthroid), she continues to have some clinical manifestations that she did not previously know were related to the hypothyroidism. Lorrie continues to tire easily, feel cold despite warmer environmental temperatures, and struggle with constipation. Alissa has found some nursing interventions through her study of hypothyroidism that may be useful to her grandmother.

Exercise 6-23: *Multiple-choice question*

When educating her grandmother on controlling her fatigue, Alissa determines that she understands the information when she states:

    A. "I should push to get all of my housework done in one block of time."

    B. "I don't want to ask for help; I need to keep pushing myself."

    C. "I need to get used to feeling tired since I will feel like this the rest of my life."

    D. "I need to space my activities so I can rest in between."

Exercise 6-24: *Multiple-choice question*

When educating Lorrie on how to maintain a normal body temperature, her granddaughter determines that she needs further instruction when she states:

    A. "I can just layer my clothing to provide more warmth."

    B. "I can use heating pads or an electric blanket when I go to bed."

    C. "I should stay away from cold, drafty areas."

    D. "I won't feel cold all the time once my medicine starts working."

Exercise 6-25: *Select all that apply*

Identify interventions designed to improve constipation:

❑ Use laxatives regularly

❑ Increase fluid intake if no restrictions

❑ Increase activity as tolerated

❑ Use enemas on a biweekly schedule

❑ Increase fiber content in diet

Answers to this chapter begin on page 231.

eResource 6-17: For more patient education information, refer to *Hypothyroidism: What Every Patient Needs to Know:* http://goo.gl/jM09p

Alissa has completed her study of hypothyroidism and educated her grandmother on her disease process, but she decides to review a little information on hyperthyroidism since she knows that this can occur as a result of ingestion of too much thyroid hormone.

Exercise 6-26: *Select all that apply*
Identify clinical manifestations associated with hyperthyroidism:

❑ Nervousness

❑ Heat intolerance

❑ Progressive weight gain

❑ Poor appetite and decreased intake

❑ Tachycardia

Exercise 6-27: *Fill-in*
Identify three atypical signs and symptoms of hyperthyroidism that the elderly patient may present:

1. _____

2. _____

3. _____

 eResource 6-18: Alissa uses Medscape on her mobile device to supplement her understanding of hyperthyroidism: [Pathway: Medscape → enter "hyperthyroidism" into the search field → review content]

Exercise 6-28: *True or false*
Identify whether the following statements about laboratory results used to diagnose hyperthyroidism are true or false:

_____ 1. TSH levels are decreased with untreated hyperthyroidism.

_____ 2. Free T4 levels are decreased with untreated hyperthyroidism.

Unfolding Case Study #38 ▨ Linda

Linda is a 58-year-old female with a medical history of hypertension, asthma, and chronic bronchitis. She has a past history of smoking one to one and a half packs of cigarettes per day for 35 years. Linda quit smoking when her asthma worsened; she has been smoke-free for 3 years now. As part of her treatment regimen, Linda has been taking prednisone 20 mg orally daily for the past 12 months. At her most recent primary care provider's (PCP) appointment, Linda expresses concern at the changes that are occurring in her body. She reports that she is putting on weight and her face has become very round. She has also noticed increasing hair growth on her face. Linda shows the nurse multiple bruises on her arms.

Exercise 6-29: *Fill-in*

Taking into consideration Linda's medical history, medications prescribed, and presenting signs and symptoms, the nurse believes that Linda has manifestations of

_____.

Exercise 6-30: *Fill-in*

Identify the three types of steroid hormones and their prototypes that are produced by the adrenal cortex:

1. _____

2. _____

3. _____

Exercise 6-31: *Short answer*

Briefly explain how the hormones secreted by the adrenal cortex are regulated through the hypothalamic-pituitary-adrenal axis.

_____

_____

_____

_____

_____

_____

Exercise 6-32: *Matching*

Match the adrenal hormone in Column A with its effects in Column B.

Column A	Column B
A. Glucocorticoids	_____ Major effects on electrolyte metabolism; long-term regulation of sodium balance
B. Mineralocorticoids	_____ Effects similar to male sex hormones; secretes small amount of estrogen
C. Sex hormones	_____ Influence glucose metabolism; inhibit the inflammatory response

eResource 6-19: To reinforce your understanding of the function of the adrenal cortex, view the following video, *Adrenal Gland Explained Clearly!*, by Dr. Roger Seheult,
- Part 1: http://youtu.be/fF_3mJV3Yh0
- Part 2: http://youtu.be/TLzqjRvqI04

Answers to this chapter begin on page 231.

Linda is seen by her PCP and diagnosed with Cushing's syndrome. She is surprised to learn that the medicine that is helping keep her asthma under control is likely the source of her new signs and symptoms. The PCP has talked to Linda about making changes to her medication regimen, but Linda is concerned about how this will impact her asthma. She has many questions about how prednisone can cause Cushing's syndrome.

Exercise 6-33: *Short answer*
Briefly explain how the use of prednisone can lead to Cushing's syndrome.

_____

_____

_____

eResource 6-20: To supplement your teaching regarding prednisone, refer to Epocrates Online: [Pathway: → http://online.epocrates.com → select the "Medication" tab → enter "Predisone" into the search field → select "patient teaching" and review content]

Exercise 6-34: *Select all that apply*
Identify other potential causes of Cushing's syndrome:

❑ Hyperplasia of the adrenal cortex

❑ Pituitary gland tumors

❑ Thyroid gland tumors

❑ Bronchogenic carcinoma

❑ Undersecretion of adrenocorticotropic hormone

eResource 6-21: To learn more about causes of Cushing's syndrome, consult the Merck Manual: [Pathway: www.merckmanuals.com → select "Merck Manual of Diagnosis and Therapy" → enter "Cushing's Syndrome" into the search field → select "Cushing's Syndrome" → select "Etiology" and review content]

Exercise 6-35: *Select all that apply*
Identify clinical manifestations associated with Cushing's syndrome:

❑ Truncal obesity

❑ Buffalo hump

❑ Hyponatremia

❑ Impaired wound healing

❑ Mood changes

❑ Hypoglycemia

❑ Osteoporosis

eResource 6-22: To learn more about the clinical presentation of Cushing's syndrome, refer to Medscape on your mobile device: [Pathway: Medscape → enter "Cushing's syndrome" into the search field → select "Clinical Presentation" and review content]

The PCP has ordered a basic metabolic panel (BMP) and an overnight dexamethasone suppression test. The nurse gives Linda instructions for the overnight dexamethasone suppression test and an appointment for follow-up in 1 week.

Exercise 6-36: *True or false*

Identify whether the following statements about diagnostic findings of Cushing's syndrome are true or false:

_____ 1. Serum sodium levels may be increased.

_____ 2. Serum glucose levels may be increased.

_____ 3. Serum potassium levels may be increased.

_____ 4. A cortisol level of greater than 5 mg/dL obtained at 8 a.m. (overnight dexamethasone suppression test) indicates that the hypothalamic-pituitary-adrenal axis is functioning properly.

eResource 6-23: To learn more about the diagnostic work-up of Cushing's syndrome, refer to Medscape on your mobile device: [Pathway: Medscape → enter "Cushing's syndrome" into the search field → select "Work-Up" → select "Laboratory Studies" and review content]

Linda returns to see her PCP 1 week later. Her cortisol level is 3.6 mg/dL. The PCP explains that her Cushing's syndrome is related to her long-term prednisone use. Linda is changed to an alternate-day dosing of prednisone to decrease the signs and symptoms associated with Cushing's syndrome. The nurse then educates Linda on other interventions to help her deal with the Cushing's syndrome.

Exercise 6-37: *Fill-in*

Identify three nursing diagnoses for the patient with Cushing's syndrome:

1. _____

2. _____

3. _____

eResource 6-24: For additional information regarding developing a nursing care plan for a client with Cushing's syndrome, refer to:
- eNurse Care Plan: http://goo.gl/UNe1j
- Nursing Hubpages: http://goo.gl/RTP6F

Answers to this chapter begin on page 231.

Exercise 6-38: *Select all that apply*
Identify interventions that decrease the risk of injury and infection and promote skin integrity:

❏ Avoid use of adhesive tape on the skin

❏ Place furniture close together to assist with ambulation

❏ Avoid exposure to others with infection

❏ Encourage moderate activity with frequent position changes

❏ Establish a protective environment that helps prevent falls

Exercise 6-39: *True or false*
Identify whether the following dietary recommendations for patients with Cushing's syndrome are true or false:

_____ 1. Select foods low in calcium and vitamin D to minimize osteoporosis

_____ 2. Select foods high in protein to minimize muscle wasting

_____ 3. Follow a low-sodium, low-carbohydrate diet to control weight gain

 eResource 6-25: For more patient education information to provide to Linda, refer to the NIH's publication "Cushing's Syndrome": http://goo.gl/UbClf

Exercise 6-40: *Multiple-choice question*
What is the nurse's best response when Linda remarks that she is so upset about her physical appearance and body changes that have occurred as a result of Cushing's syndrome?

A. "Unfortunately, you can't control these signs and symptoms."

B. "I know how you must be feeling about all these changes."

C. "As the Cushing's syndrome is treated, the physical changes will eventually disappear."

D. "Perhaps you need to talk to someone about your concerns."

Exercise 6-41: *Multiple-choice question*
When educating Linda on the correct administration of prednisone, the nurse determines that she understands the information when she states:

A. "Since I am on prednisone only once every other day, it does not matter what time I take the medication."

B. "It is best to take my prednisone at 8 a.m. on my scheduled days."

C. "I am less likely to have signs and symptoms of Cushing's syndrome if I take my prednisone from 4 p.m. to 8 p.m. on my scheduled days."

D. "I should divide the dose to take it twice a day on my scheduled days."

Answers to this chapter begin on page 231.

Exercise 6-42: *Short answer*

Briefly explain why patients prescribed corticosteroid medications should never abruptly stop taking them.

_____

_____

_____

 eResource 6-26: To reinforce patient teaching regarding prednisone, its indication and effects, on your mobile device, consult:

- Medscape: [Pathway: Medscape → enter "Prednisone" into the search field → review content]
- Skyscape's RxDrugs: [Pathway: RxDrugs → enter "Prednisone" into the search field → review content]
- Epocrates: [Pathway: Epocrates → enter "Prednisone" into the search field → review content]

Answers to this chapter begin on page 231.

Answers

Exercise 6-1: *Select all that apply*

Identify risk factors commonly associated with diabetes mellitus:

- ☒ **Obesity—YES**
- ❏ Age under 45 years—NO, usually occurs with ages over 45 years.
- ❏ Caucasian race—NO, higher incidence with African Americans, Hispanics, Native Americans, Asian Americans, and Pacific Islanders.
- ☒ **Family history—YES**
- ☒ **History of gestational diabetes—YES**
- ☒ **History of delivering babies over 9 pounds—YES**

Exercise 6-2: *Multiple-choice question*

The nurse educating Jenny on type 2 diabetes determines that she understands the information when she states:

A. "I am not producing any insulin because of a problem with my immune system."—NO, this occurs with type 1 diabetes.

B. "I will need to take insulin for the rest of my life."—NO, type 2 diabetics usually begin treatment with dietary changes and oral medications.

C. **"I'm not making enough insulin or my body isn't as sensitive to it."—YES**

D. "I won't need to make any dietary changes if I take my medicine."—NO, dietary changes are the first line of treatment with type 2 diabetes.

Exercise 6-3: *Matching*

Match the type of diabetes in Column A with its typical characteristics in Column B. Answers in Column A can be used more than once.

Column A		Column B
A. Type 1 diabetes	**A**	Onset is usually below 30 years old
B. Type 2 diabetes	**A**	Patient is often thin at time of diagnosis
	B	Treated with diet, exercise, and oral agents
	B	Patient is often obese at time of diagnosis
	A	Antibodies are present in the body
	A	Patients require insulin for life

Exercise 6-4: *Select all that apply*
Identify common clinical manifestations associated with diabetes mellitus:

☒ **Polyuria—YES, urination increases related to increased glucose levels.**

❑ Decreased appetite—NO, polyphagia (increased appetite) results from the catabolic state that occurs with insulin deficiency.

❑ Decreased fluid intake—NO, polydipsia (increased thirst) occurs related to excess fluid loss.

☒ **Vision changes—YES**

☒ **Fatigue—YES**

Exercise 6-5: *Short answer*
Briefly explain how a HgbA1C is used to evaluate blood glucose compared to a random blood glucose level. **A random blood glucose tests the glucose level at the point that the blood is drawn. A HgbA1C reflects average blood glucose levels over a period of 2 to 3 months. When blood glucose is elevated for a period of time, the glucose attaches to the hemoglobin for the life of the red blood cell (approximately 120 days). A HgbA1C is a good indicator of glycemic control.**

Exercise 6-6: *Fill-in*
Identify three ways in which metformin acts to maintain normal blood glucose levels:
1. **Decreases glucose production by the liver**
2. **Decreases intestinal absorption of glucose**
3. **Increases sensitivity to insulin**

Exercise 6-7: *Fill-in*
For obese patients who are diabetic, the key to treatment is: **weight loss.**

Exercise 6-8: *Fill-in*
Identify the food groups that are part of the Exchange List system and give one example of a specific food within each group:
1. **Bread/starches—bread, cereal, corn, crackers**
2. **Fruits—apples, cherries, peaches, fruit juice**
3. **Milk—milks, yogurts**
4. **Meat—beef, pork, eggs, cheese, fish**
5. **Nonstarchy vegetables—broccoli, cucumbers, tomatoes, onions**
6. **Sweets, desserts, and other carbohydrates—cake, pies, brownies, candy**
7. **Fats—nuts, mayonnaise, salad dressing, margarine**
8. **Free foods—sugar-free gelatin, diet sodas, tea, mustard, garlic**

Exercise 6-9: *True of false*

Identify whether the following statements about nutrition in the diabetic patient are true or false:

True   1. Soluble fiber lowers blood glucose levels by slowing the rate of glucose absorption from these foods.

True   2. Alcohol used in combination with chlorpropamide (Diabinese) may cause facial flushing, warmth, nausea, and vomiting.

False   3. Nutritive sweeteners have no effect on blood glucose levels.

Exercise 6-10: *Multiple-choice question*

The nurse educating Jenny on exercise determines that she needs further instruction when she states:

A. "Exercise will lower my blood glucose level."—NO

B. "I should try to exercise at the same time each day."—NO

C. "Walking is generally a safe form of exercise."—NO

D. "I should exercise more when my glucose levels are more than 250 mg/dL."— YES, exercise further increases the release of glucagon, growth hormone, and catecholamines, which will further increase blood glucose levels.

Exercise 6-11: *Select all that apply*

Identify other circumstances in which more frequent testing is recommended:

☐ Missing a mealtime—NO, unless symptoms of hypoglycemia.

☒ **Symptoms of hypoglycemia—YES**

☒ **Changes in medications—YES**

☒ **During periods of increased stress—YES, stress can increase blood glucose levels.**

☒ **Times of illness—YES, blood glucose levels can increase with illness.**

Exercise 6-12: *Matching*

Match the medication in Column A with its drug classification and action in Column B.

Column A		Column B
A. chlorpropamide (Diabinese)	**D**	Alpha-glucosidase inhibitor; delays intestinal absorption of complex carbs
B. glipizide (Glucotrol)	**A**	First-generation sulfonylurea; stimulates beta cells of the pancreas to secrete insulin
C. metformin (Glucophage)	**E**	Nonsulfonylurea insulin secretagogue; stimulates the pancreas to secrete insulin
D. acarbose (Precose)	**B**	Second-generation sulfonylurea; stimulates beta cells of the pancreas to secrete insulin
E. nateglinide (Starlix)	**C**	Biguanide; inhibits production of glucose by the liver

Exercise 6-13: *Multiple-choice question*
The nurse educating Jenny on hypoglycemia determines that she understands the information when she states:
A. "I won't get hypoglycemic when I am only taking metformin."—NO, hypoglycemia can still occur while taking oral agents.
B. "If I feel my blood sugar dropping, I will eat some chocolate candy."—NO, avoid treating hypoglycemia with high-calorie, high-fat dessert foods.
C. **"My family should be educated on how to help me if I become hypoglycemic."— YES, so they can assist if the patient is becoming confused or impaired.**
D. "Hypoglycemia most often occurs 1 hour after meals."—NO, hypoglycemia usually occurs before meals or when meals are missed.

Exercise 6-14: *Fill-in*
Identify the macrovascular and microvascular complications that can occur with diabetes:

Macrovascular	Microvascular
1. **Coronary artery disease**	1. **Retinopathy**
2. **Cerebrovascular disease**	2. **Nephropathy**
3. **Peripheral vascular disease**	

Exercise 6-15: *Select all that apply*
Identify foot care techniques recommended for diabetic patients:
☒ **Assess feet daily—YES, look for cuts, blisters, or reddened areas.**
❑ Lotion the feet, especially between the toes—NO, not between the toes.
❑ Use hot water for soaking the feet—NO, feet should not be soaked; wash only in warm water.
☒ **Trim toenails straight across—YES, to avoid cutting surrounding skin.**
☒ **Never walk barefoot—YES, to protect the feet.**

Exercise 6-16: *Select all that apply*
Identify the hormones released by the thyroid gland:
☒ **Thyroxine (T4)—YES**
❑ Thyroid-stimulating hormone (TSH)—NO, this is released by the anterior pituitary gland.
☒ **Triiodothyronine (T3)—YES**
☒ **Calcitonin—YES**
❑ Antidiuretic hormone (ADH)—NO, this is released by the posterior pituitary gland.

Exercise 6-17: *Fill-in*

Essential for the synthesis of thyroid hormones, **iodine** is obtained through diet.

Exercise 6-18: *Short answer*

Briefly explain how the release of thyroid hormone is regulated in the body.

Thyroid-stimulating hormone (TSH) regulates the release of triiodothyronine (T3) and thyroxine (T4) through a negative feedback mechanism. For example, if the level of thyroid hormone in the body decreases, TSH from the anterior pituitary gland will be released, which in turn causes more T3 and T4 to be released from the thyroid gland. As the level of thyroid hormone increases, TSH release will decrease, which in turn slows the release of T3 and T4.

Exercise 6-19: *Fill-in*

Identify three common signs and symptoms that may indicate an endocrine disorder:

1. **Change in energy level/fatigue**
2. **Change in tolerance to heat or cold**
3. **Change in sexual function or sexual characteristics**
4. **Change in mood, memory, or ability to concentrate**
5. **Altered sleep patterns**
6. **Weight changes**

Exercise 6-20: *Select all that apply*

Identify clinical manifestations associated with hypothyroidism:

❏ Weight loss—NO, weight gain usually occurs.

☒ **Fatigue—YES, may be extreme.**

☒ **Irritability—YES, but may become subdued as the condition progresses.**

☒ **Hair loss—YES**

❏ Increased pulse—NO, pulse rate slows with severe hypothyroidism.

☒ **Feeling cold in a warm environment—YES**

Exercise 6-21: *Matching*

Match the laboratory test in Column A with its description and normal value in Column B.

Column A	Column B	
A. TSH	**C**	70% is protein-bound; normal is 5 to 11 mcg/dL
B. T3	**D**	Direct measurement of unbound thyroxine; normal is 0.8 to 2.7 ng/dL
C. T4		
D. Free T4	**A**	Best screening test for thyroid function; normal is 0.4 to 4.2 mIU/L
	B	More accurate indicator of hyperthyroidism; normal is 70 to 204 ng/dL

Exercise 6-22: *True or false*

Identify whether the following statements about thyroid hormone replacement therapy are true or false:

True   1. TSH levels are used for monitoring the effectiveness of thyroid hormone replacement and in making dosage adjustments of the medications.

True   2. Signs of overdose are manifested as hyperthyroidism (tachycardia, weight loss, nervousness, and/or chest pain).

False   3. Thyroid hormone replacement is only needed until symptoms subside; the medication can then be discontinued.

Exercise 6-23: *Multiple-choice question*

When educating her grandmother on controlling her fatigue, Alissa determines that she understands the information when she states:

A. "I should push to get all of my housework done in one block of time."—NO, this will overtire her, and likely make her feel even more fatigued.

B. "I don't want to ask for help; I need to keep pushing myself."—NO, this will overtire her; it is okay to ask for help.

C. "I need to get used to feeling tired since I will feel like this the rest of my life."—NO, the fatigue should lessen as the medication becomes therapeutic and her thyroid levels return to normal.

D. "I need to space my activities so I can rest in between."—YES, this allows her to participate in activities while allowing for adequate rest.

Exercise 6-24: *Multiple-choice question*

When educating Lorrie on how to maintain a normal body temperature, her granddaughter determines that she needs further instruction when she states:

A. "I can just layer my clothing to provide more warmth."—NO

B. "I can use heating pads or an electric blanket when I go to bed."—YES, these should not be used until hypothyroidism is corrected; peripheral vasodilation and vascular collapse can occur.

C. "I should stay away from cold, drafty areas."—NO

D. "I won't feel cold all the time once my medicine starts working."—NO

Exercise 6-25: *Select all that apply*

Identify interventions designed to improve constipation:

☐ Use laxatives regularly—NO, this increases dependence on elimination aids.

☒ **Increase fluid intake if no restrictions—YES, this softens stool.**

☒ **Increase activity as tolerated—YES, this promotes evacuation of stool.**

☐ Use enemas on a biweekly schedule—NO, this increases dependence on elimination aids.

☒ **Increase fiber content in diet—YES, this increases stool bulk leading to more frequent bowel movements.**

Exercise 6-26: *Select all that apply*

Identify clinical manifestations associated with hyperthyroidism:

☒ **Nervousness—YES**

☒ **Heat intolerance—YES**

❑ Progressive weight gain—NO, progressive weight loss occurs.

❑ Poor appetite and decreased intake—NO, there is increased appetite and food intake.

☒ **Tachycardia—YES, the patient may also experience palpitations.**

Exercise 6-27: *Fill-in*

Identify three atypical signs and symptoms of hyperthyroidism that the elderly patient may present:

1. **Anorexia and weight loss**
2. **Isolated atrial fibrillation**
3. **New or worsening angina**
4. **New or worsening heart failure**

Exercise 6-28: *True or false*

Identify whether the following statements about laboratory results used to diagnose hyperthyroidism are true or false:

True   1. TSH levels are decreased with untreated hyperthyroidism.

False   2. Free T4 levels are decreased with untreated hyperthyroidism.

Exercise 6-29: *Fill-in*

Taking into consideration Linda's medical history, medications prescribed, and presenting signs and symptoms, the nurse believes that Linda has manifestations of **Cushing's syndrome.**

Exercise 6-30: *Fill-in*

Identify the three types of steroid hormones and their prototypes that are produced by the adrenal cortex:

1. **Glucocorticoids—hydrocortisone**
2. **Mineralocorticoids—aldosterone**
3. **Sex hormones—androgens**

Exercise 6-31: *Short answer*

Briefly explain how the hormones secreted by the adrenal cortex are regulated through the hypothalamic-pituitary-adrenal axis.

The hypothalamic-pituitary-adrenal axis uses a negative feedback mechanism. When increased levels of adrenal hormone are needed, the hypothalamus secretes corticotropin-releasing hormone (CRH), which in turn stimulates the pituitary gland to secrete adrenocorticotropic hormone (ACTH), which in turn stimulates

the adrenal cortex to release glucocorticoids. When there are sufficient levels of adrenal hormones, secretion of CRH and ACTH is inhibited.

Exercise 6-32: *Matching*
Match the adrenal hormone in Column A with its effects in Column B.

Column A	Column B
A. Glucocorticoids	__B__ Major effects on electrolyte metabolism; long-term regulation of sodium balance
B. Mineralocorticoids	__C__ Effects similar to male sex hormones; secretes small amount of estrogen
C. Sex hormones	__A__ Influence glucose metabolism; inhibit the inflammatory response

Exercise 6-33: *Short answer*
Briefly explain how the use of prednisone can lead to Cushing's syndrome.
Long-term use of oral corticosteroid medications, such as prednisone, and especially in higher doses, can cause high levels of cortisol in the body. These sustained high levels of cortisol can cause the manifestations associated with Cushing's syndrome.

Exercise 6-34: *Select all that apply*
Identify potential causes of Cushing's syndrome:

☒ **Hyperplasia of the adrenal cortex—YES, this can cause overproduction of corticosteroids.**

☒ **Pituitary gland tumors—YES, if the tumor produces increased amounts of ACTH.**

❑ Thyroid gland tumors—NO

☒ **Bronchogenic carcinoma—YES, this malignancy can cause ectopic production of ACTH.**

❑ Undersecretion of ACTH—NO, this would lead to Addison's disease.

Exercise 6-35: *Select all that apply*
Identify clinical manifestations associated with Cushing's syndrome:

☒ **Truncal obesity—YES**

☒ **Buffalo hump—YES, this is a fatty area in the neck and supraclavicular areas.**

❑ Hyponatremia—NO, sodium retention occurs.

☒ **Impaired wound healing—YES, and increased susceptibility to infections.**

☒ **Mood changes—YES, distress and depression are common.**

❑ Hypoglycemia—NO, hyperglycemia occurs.

☒ **Osteoporosis—YES, kyphosis and compression fractures may occur.**

Exercise 6-36: *True or false*
Identify whether the following statements about diagnostic findings of Cushing's syndrome are true or false:

True   1. Serum sodium levels may be increased.

True   2. Serum glucose levels may be increased.

False   3. Serum potassium levels may be increased.

False   4. A cortisol level of greater than 5 mg/dL obtained at 8 a.m. (overnight dexamethasone suppression test) indicates that the hypothalamic-pituitary-adrenal axis is functioning properly.

Exercise 6-37: *Fill-in*
Identify three nursing diagnoses for the patient with Cushing's syndrome:

1. **Disturbed body image related to altered physical appearance**
2. **Disturbed thought processes related to mood swings and irritability**
3. **Impaired skin integrity related to thin, fragile skin**
4. **Self-care deficit related to weakness and fatigue**
5. **Risk for injury related to weakness**
6. **Risk for infection related to inflammatory response**

Exercise 6-38: *Select all that apply*
Identify interventions that decrease the risk of injury and infection and promote skin integrity:

☒ **Avoid use of adhesive tape on the skin—YES, this can irritate and tear fragile skin.**

❏ Place furniture close together to assist with ambulation—NO, this increases the risk of bumping into sharp edges and tearing fragile skin.

☒ **Avoid exposure to others with infection—YES, patients with Cushing's syndrome are more susceptible to infections.**

☒ **Encourage moderate activity with frequent position changes—YES, this prevents complications from immobility.**

☒ **Establish a protective environment that helps prevent falls—YES, this prevents injury to bones, soft tissues, and skin.**

Exercise 6-39: *True or false*
Identify whether the following dietary recommendations for patients with Cushing's syndrome are true or false:

False   1. Select foods low in calcium and vitamin D to minimize osteoporosis.

True   2. Select foods high in protein to minimize muscle wasting.

True   3. Follow a low sodium, low carbohydrate diet to control weight gain.

Exercise 6-40: *Multiple-choice question*
What is the nurse's best response when Linda remarks that she is so upset about her physical appearance and body changes that have occurred as a result of Cushing's syndrome?
A. "Unfortunately, you can't control these signs and symptoms."—NO, this is not a helpful response.
B. "I know how you must be feeling about all these changes."—NO, no one can know how another person feels.
C. "As the Cushing's syndrome is treated, the physical changes will eventually disappear."—YES, with successful treatment, signs and symptoms of the syndrome disappear.
D. "Perhaps you need to talk to someone about your concerns."—NO, the patient is sharing her feelings with the nurse; it is important not to dismiss her

Exercise 6-41: *Multiple-choice question*
When educating Linda on the correct administration of prednisone, the nurse determines that she understands the information when she states:
A. "Since I am on prednisone only once every other day, it does not matter what time I take the medication."—NO
B. "It is best to take my prednisone at 8 a.m. on my scheduled days."—YES, this is in keeping with the natural secretion of cortisol in the body.
C. "I am less likely to have signs and symptoms of Cushing's syndrome if I take my prednisone from 4 p.m. to 8 p.m. on my scheduled days."—NO, signs and symptoms are more likely to occur if dosages are taken between 4 p.m. and 6 a.m., when cortisol levels are normally low.
D. "I should divide the dose to take it twice a day on my scheduled days."—NO, this increases the risk of signs and symptoms of Cushing's syndrome.

Exercise 6-42: *Short answer*
Briefly explain why patients prescribed corticosteroid medications should never abruptly stop taking them.
When patients are taking corticosteroids, the action of the medication suppresses the natural function of the adrenal cortex. If corticosteroids are stopped abruptly, adrenal insufficiency may occur. Dosages should be tapered gradually to allow normal adrenal function to return.

7

Nursing Care of the Patient With Immunological Disease

Rhonda M. Brogdon

Unfolding Case Study #39 ▪ Eva

Eva is a 25-year-old patient who presents to an outpatient clinic complaining of night sweats and fatigue. She reported nausea and vomiting for 3 days, decreased appetite, diarrhea, white-colored lesions on her inner cheeks (thrush), and abdominal pain rated 5 on a scale of 0 to 10, with 10 being the highest pain. She has a low-grade temperature of 100.8°F, pulse of 98, respirations of 22, and blood pressure of 126/70. Her medical history is positive for allergies and intravenous (IV) drug use, and she is sexually active. She states, "I don't always have protected sex."

Exercise 7-1: *Fill-in*
The nurse suspects a possible diagnosis of:

_____.

To confirm the diagnosis, the primary care provider (PCP) orders a CD4+ count, enzyme-linked immunosorbent assay (ELISA), and a Western blot test.

Exercise 7-2: *Fill-in*
What is the significance of the CD4+ count? _____

_____

What is the significance of the Western blot test? _____

_____

What is the significance of an ELISA? _____

_____

The ELISA came back positive. Her CD4+ count was 189 cells/mm³ and the Western blot confirmed the diagnosis.

Exercise 7-3: *Multiple-choice question*

What is the accepted range for the CD4+ count?

    A. 100 to 5,000 cells/mm³

    B. 500 to 1,000 cells/mm³

    C. 300 to 5,000 cells/mm³

    D. 800 to 1,000 cells/mm³

Exercise 7-4: *Multiple-choice question*

The nurse knows that CD4+ lymphocytes are also called:

    A. R-cells

    B. D-cells

    C. T-cells

    D. J-cells

Exercise 7-5: *Fill-in*

What is the function of CD4+ lymphocytes? _____

_____

 eResource 7-1: For more information about HIV testing, consult Medscape on your mobile device:
- Overview: [Pathway: Medscape → enter "HIV" into the search field → select "HIV Testing Overview" and review content]
- HIV Antibody Testing: [Pathway: Medscape → enter "HIV" into the search field → select "HIV Antibody Testing" and review content]
- Pathophysiology: [Pathway: Medscape → enter "HIV" into the search field → select "HIV disease" → select "pathophysiology" and review content]

The PCP has notified Eva that she is positive for HIV (human immunodeficiency virus) and AIDS (acquired immunodeficiency syndrome). Eva starts crying and says, "How do I have both?"

Exercise 7-6: *Fill-in*

How does the primary care provider explain the differences between HIV and AIDS to Eva?

HIV is _____

_____

AIDS is _____

_____

 eResource 7-2: To learn more about HIV and AIDS, Eva views the following videos:
- *Understanding HIV and AIDS (HIV #1)*: http://youtu.be/P91nIGt1axs
- *When HIV Becomes AIDS (HIV #2)*: http://youtu.be/68I7JlVhuhY
- *HIV/AIDS Myths: Ten More Myths About HIV and AIDS*: http://youtu.be/bURqMwLWV40

Answers to this chapter begin on page 255.

Exercise 7-7: *Fill-in*

What two risk factors predisposed Eva to HIV/AIDS?

1. _____

2. _____

> **eResource 7-3:** To learn more about the risk factors for HIV/AIDS, consult Epocrates Online: [Pathway: → http://online.epocrates.com → select the "diseases" tab → enter "HIV" into the search field → review content related to "risks"]

Exercise 7-8: *Fill-in*

What signs and symptoms did Eva present that gave the suspicion of HIV/AIDS?

1. _____

2. _____

3. _____

4. _____

5. _____

6. _____

7. _____

> **eResource 7-4:** To learn more about the clinical presentation of HIV/AIDS, consult the Merck Manual: [Pathway: www.merckmanuals.com → select "Merck Manual of Diagnosis and Therapy" → enter "HIV" into the search field → select "Human Immunodeficiency Virus (HIV)" → select "Symptoms and Signs" and review content]

The PCP explains to Eva that there are three stages of HIV infection.

Exercise 7-9: *Matching*

Match the stage of HIV in Column A with its definition in Column B.

Column A	Column B
A. Stage 1: Primary HIV infection	_____ Individuals are free from symptoms of HIV; levels of HIV are low in blood
B. Stage 2: Asymptomatic HIV	_____ Experience flu-like symptoms; lasts a few weeks
C. Stage 3: AIDS	_____ Diagnosed as having AIDS; cannot return to stage of HIV

Exercise 7-10: *Fill-in*

What stage of infection is Eva experiencing?_____

Eva has been admitted into the hospital. She had a white blood count of 3,000 mm^3 and her creatinine clearance was within range of 125 mL/min. The PCP has ordered Megace 40 mg twice a day by mouth, daily measurement of weight, high-calorie, protein-rich diet in six small meals daily once nausea and vomiting subside, intravenous fluids of normal saline at 150 mL/hr, acyclovir 350 mg IV every 8 hours, Epogen 100 units/kg subcutaneously three times a week, zidovudine 100 mg every 4 hours by mouth, vancomycin 800 mg IV every 6 hours, Neupogen 300 mcg subcutaneously daily, Diflucan 200 mg daily for 7 days, Phenergan 12.5 mg IV every 4 hours as needed for nausea, Imodium for diarrhea as needed, and a chest x-ray.

Exercise 7-11: *Calculation*

Calculate how many mL of Neupogen will be given subcutaneously. The vial is labeled 300 mcg/mL.

Exercise 7-12: *Calculation*

Calculate how many mL of Epogen will be given subcutaneously to Eva who weighs 120 pounds. The vial is labeled 4000 units/mL.

 eResource 7-5: To verify your calculations for weight conversion, consult Skyscape's Archimedes on your mobile device: [Pathway: Archimedes → enter "weight conversion" into the search field → enter patient data]

Exercise 7-13: *Calculation*

Calculate how many mL/hr to set the IV pump to infuse vancomycin 500 mg. It is supplied as a 1-g vial to be reconstituted with 10 mL normal saline solution and further diluted in 100 mL D5W to infuse over 60 minutes.

 eResource 7-6: To verify your calculations, consult Skyscape's Archimedes on your mobile device: [Pathway: Archimedes → enter "IV" into the search field → select "IV Calc: infuse a volume" and enter medication order data]

Exercise 7-14: *Select all that apply*

What teaching(s) by the nurse will benefit Eva once she is discharged home?

❏ Complying with anti-retroviral medications

❏ Referral to AIDS support groups

❏ Encourage use of coping mechanisms

❏ Alternate activity with rest periods

❏ Maintain a well-balanced diet

❏ Follow-up with CD4+ count

❏ Reporting of signs and symptoms of infection not needed

Answers to this chapter begin on page 255.

eResource 7-7: For more information to provide patient teaching, refer to:
- *CDC's Living With HIV/AIDS:* http://goo.gl/9Toqe
- *Coping With HIV and AIDS*: http://goo.gl/zVvqH

Exercise 7-15: *Fill-in*
Why will the primary care provider order another CD4+ count?

_____

_____

Exercise 7-16: *Select all that apply*
Based upon Eva's diagnosis and assessment findings, what nursing diagnoses are pertinent in her care?
- ❑ Risk for infection
- ❑ Imbalanced nutrition: more than body requirements
- ❑ Ineffective coping
- ❑ Fatigue/activity intolerance
- ❑ Imbalanced nutrition: less than body requirements

 eResource 7-8: For more information regarding nursing care of patients with HIV/AIDS, refer to:
- Nursing Care of Patients with HIV/AIDS: http://goo.gl/mwD8e
- University of California–San Francisco's *HIV InSite*: http://goo.gl/CYWYe

Unfolding Case Study #40 ▓ Mabel

Mabel is a 70-year-old patient who was diagnosed with rheumatoid arthritis at the age of 50. She has complained of increasing pain in her hands, wrists, shoulders, and knees; in addition, she complained of morning stiffness that hinders her activities. Mabel rates her pain a 6 on a numerical scale of 1 to 10, with 10 being the highest level of pain. She has a medical history of hysterectomy, seven vaginal births, and cholecystectomy, and a family history of rheumatoid arthritis and breast cancer. Mabel has been taking Enbrel 50 mg/weekly subcutaneously for 3 years, and she takes over-the-counter ibuprofen 220 mg as needed and naproxen 220 mg as needed to help reduce her pain.

 eResource 7-9: To reinforce your understanding of Mabel's current medications and their effects, consult Epocrates on your mobile device: [Pathway: Epocrates → enter "Enbrel" into the search field and review content. Repeat with "ibuprofen" and "naproxen"]

Exercise 7-17: *Fill-in*
What is rheumatoid arthritis? _____

_____

eResource 7-10: To learn more about rheumatoid arthritis, consult the following:
- Medscape on your mobile device [Pathway: Medscape → enter "rheumatoid" into the search field → select "Rheumatoid Arthritis" and review content under "overview"]
- Merck Manual online [Pathway: www.merckmanuals.com → select "Merck Manual of Diagnosis and Therapy" → enter "rheumatoid" into the search field → select "Rheumatoid Arthritis" → review content]

Exercise 7-18: *Fill-in*

The hallmark symptom in rheumatoid arthritis is _____.

eResource 7-11: To learn more about the clinical presentation of rheumatoid arthritis, refer to Medscape on your mobile device: [Pathway. Medscape → enter "rheumatoid" into the search field → select "rheumatoid arthritis" and review content under "Clinical Presentation"]

Exercise 7-19: *Select all that apply*

What are risk factors for rheumatoid arthritis?
- ❏ Female gender
- ❏ Age 30 to 50 years
- ❏ Family history
- ❏ Smoking
- ❏ Diet high in protein

eResource 7-12: To learn more about the risk factors associated with rheumatoid arthritis, refer to Epocrates Online: [Pathway: http://online .epocrates.com → select the "diseases" tab → enter "rheumatoid arthritis" into the search field → select "Rheumatoid Arthritis" and review content under "risk factors." Also be sure to review "etiology"]

The primary care provider (PCP) has ordered blood testing to evaluate the extent of Mabel's rheumatoid arthritis. He has ordered a rheumatoid factor (RF) antibody, erythrocyte sedimentation rate (ESR) test, antinuclear antibody (ANA) titer, and a white blood cell (WBC) count.

Exercise 7-20: *Fill-in*

What do these tests tell us as they relate to rheumatoid arthritis?

1. RF antibody _____

2. ESR _____

3. ANA titer _____

4. WBC count _____

The PCP has also ordered diagnostic imaging to evaluate Mabel's rheumatoid arthritis.

Answers to this chapter begin on page 255.

eResource 7-13: To learn more about the diagnostic work-up ordered for Mabel, refer to:

- Epocrates Online: [Pathway: http://online.epocrates.com → select "diseases" tab → enter "rheumatoid" into the search field → select "Rheumatoid Arthritis" → review content under "Diagnosis"]
- Merck Manual: [Pathway: www.merckmanuals.com → select "Merck Manual of Diagnosis and Therapy" → enter "rheumatoid" into the search field → select "Rheumatoid Arthritis" → review content under "Diagnosis"]

Exercise 7-21: *Matching*

Match the diagnostic imaging test in Column A to its procedure in Column B.

Column A	Column B
A. Dual energy x-ray absorptiometry	_____ Detects bone erosions in hands in rheumatoid arthritis
B. Ultrasound	_____ Monitors inflammatory activity
C. Magnetic resonance imaging	_____ Detects early bone loss in rheumatoid arthritis

Exercise 7-22: *Multiple-choice question*

What is the priority nursing diagnosis for Mabel based upon the nurse's assessment?

    A. Fatigue

    B. Pain

    C. Disturbed body image

    D. Impaired physical mobility

The PCP has made changes in Mabel's medications to help reduce the inflammatory process of her rheumatoid arthritis. He has added Plaquenil 400 mg once a day, prednisone 60 mg once a day, and Humira 40 mg subcutaneously every week to her regimen. The PCP discontinued Enbrel and ibuprofen and continued naproxen 220 mg every 4 hours as needed for pain.

Exercise 7-23: *Fill-in*

Name three side effects of Plaquenil:

    1. _____

    2. _____

    3. _____

Exercise 7-24: *Fill-in*

Name three side effects of Humira:

    1. _____

    2. _____

    3. _____

Answers to this chapter begin on page 255.

eResource 7-14: To reinforce your understanding of the newly prescribed medications, refer to the following resources on your mobile device:

- Epocrates: [Pathway: Epocrates → enter "Plaquenil" into the search field and review information. Repeat with "Humira" and "Prednisone"]
- Skyscape's RxDrugs: [Pathway: RxDrugs → enter "Plaquenil" into the search field and review information. Repeat with "Humira" and "Prednisone"]
- Medscape: [Pathway: Medscape → enter "Plaquenil" into the search field and review information. Repeat with "Humira" and "Prednisone"]

Exercise 7-25: *Multiple-choice question*

Mabel needs further discharge teaching when she says:

- A. "I am to pace my activities by resting for 5 to 10 minutes."
- B. "I am to take my prescribed medications as directed."
- C. "I can take a hot shower or bath to reduce the need for pain medication."
- D. "I don't have to watch my weight with rheumatoid arthritis."

 eResource 7-15: For additional information to support discharge teaching, review the following information:

- National Institutes of Health's Handout on Health: *Rheumatoid Arthritis*: http://goo.gl/Kb0Wd
- MedlinePlus's Interactive tutorial, *Rheumatoid Arthritis*: http://goo.gl/o2sT5

Unfolding Case Study #41 ▮ Georgia

Georgia is a 55-year-old patient who loves to work in her yard. She is experiencing daily joint stiffness and pain with minimal exertion. Georgia's joint stiffness and pain occur in her knees, hip, and lower back. Her pain is a 5 on a numerical scale of 0 to 10, with 10 being the highest pain level. Georgia stated that her pain occurs with activity and improves when she rests. She states that her muscle strength has declined, and it has become harder to perform activities of daily living. She takes Tylenol 650 mg for her discomfort every 4 hours as needed. Georgia's medical history is positive for two vaginal births and a urinary tract infection.

Exercise 7-26: *Fill-in*

Georgia's signs and symptoms are indicative of _____.

Exercise 7-27: *Fill-in*

What differentiates this disease process from rheumatoid arthritis?

_____

_____

Answers to this chapter begin on page 255.

eResource 7-16: To learn more about the clinical presentation of osteoarthritis, refer to:
- Medscape: [Pathway: Medscape → enter "Osteoarthritis" into the search field → review content under "clinical presentation"]
- View MelinePlus's video, *Osteoarthritis*: http://goo.gl/mJPKA

Exercise 7-28: *Select all that apply*

Identify some risk factors for osteoarthritis:

- ❑ Age
- ❑ Decreased muscle strength
- ❑ Obesity
- ❑ Genetic predisposition
- ❑ Hypertension

 eResource 7-17: To learn more about risk factors associated with osteoarthritis, refer to:
- Epocrates Online: [Pathway: http://online.epocrates.com → select the "diseases" tab → enter "osteoarthritis" into the search field and review content under "risk factors"]
- Centers for Disease Control and Prevention (CDC) Risk Factors: http://goo.gl/i0oG4

Exercise 7-29: *Select all that apply*

The nurse has assessed nodules on Georgia's hands. The nurse knows that the following type(s) of nodes are easily recognizable signs of osteoarthritis:

- ❑ Heberden's nodes
- ❑ Wilmer's nodes
- ❑ Bouchard's nodes
- ❑ Lymph nodes

 eResource 7-18: For more information regarding the recognizable signs and symptoms associated with osteoarthritis, refer to:
- Medscape: [Pathway: Medscape → enter "osteoarthritis" into the search field → read "physical examination" under the "clinical presentation" tab]
- Merck Manual: [Pathway: www.merckmanuals.com → select "Merck Manual of Diagnosis and Therapy" → enter "osteoarthritis" into the search field → select "osteoarthritis"→ select "symptoms & signs" and review content]

Georgia was given ketorolac (Toradol) 10 mg IV for her pain. Georgia stated, "My pain is a lot better."

 eResource 7-19: To reinforce your understanding of the effects of Toradol, refer to the following resources on your mobile device:
- Epocrates: [Pathway: Epocrates → enter "Toradol" into the search field and review information]

Answers to this chapter begin on page 255.

■ Skyscape's RxDrugs [Pathway: RxDrugs → enter "Toradol" into the search field and review information]

■ Medscape: [Pathway: Medscape → enter "Toradol" into the search field and review information]

The nurse teaches Georgia alternative methods she can use to reduce pain or discomfort in her joints.

Exercise 7-30: *Select all that apply*
What alternative methods can be utilized to reduce pain and discomfort of the joints?

❑ Moist heat to joints

❑ Massage of joints

❑ Adequate rest after activities

❑ Gentle range-of-motion exercises

❑ Proper body mechanics

eResource 7-20: For supplemental information regarding alternative methods for pain management, refer to the CDC website: http://goo.gl/3Jijk

Exercise 7-31: *Select all that apply*
Georgia complained of pain and a decrease in her activities due to the osteoarthritis. Based on this assessment, what are the two top nursing diagnoses for Georgia?

❑ Pain

❑ Activity intolerance

❑ Disturbed body image

❑ Impaired skin integrity

eResource 7-21: For more information regarding developing a nursing care plan for Georgia's pain and activity intolerance, refer to NANDA Nursing Interventions:
■ Activity Intolerance: http://goo.gl/p9bBT
■ Pain (Acute/Chronic) related to Osteoarthritis: http://goo.gl/XHfZv

Exercise 7-32: *Fill-in*
Identify which characteristics are indicative of osteoarthritis or rheumatoid arthritis:

Heberden's nodes _____

Progressive deterioration of articular cartilage _____

Pain occurs with activity _____

Autoimmune response _____

Systemic response _____

Unfolding Case Study #42 ▒ Roberta

Roberta is a 30-year-old patient admitted into the hospital with complaints of weakness and malaise and a butterfly rash over her nose and cheeks. She has noted some hair loss (alopecia), joint inflammation, and sensitivity to light. Roberta has a low-grade fever of 100.3°F, blood pressure of 138/88, pulse of 90, and respirations of 20. Roberta has a medical history of one vaginal birth, allergies, and a tonsillectomy.

Exercise 7-33: *Select all that apply*
What sign and symptoms in Roberta's assessment indicate a diagnosis of systemic lupus erythematosus (SLE)?

- ❏ Butterfly rash
- ❏ Weakness
- ❏ Malaise
- ❏ Low-grade fever
- ❏ Joint inflammation
- ❏ Tonsillectomy

ⓔ **eResource 7-22:** For more information regarding SLE, refer to Medscape on your mobile device: [Pathway: Medscape → enter "lupus" into the search field → select "Systemic Lupus Erythematosus (SLE)" and review information under "Clinical Presentation"]

Exercise 7-34: *Multiple-choice question*
Roberta does not understand lupus and asks the nurse what caused her to have this disease. The nurse explains to her that:

- A. Lupus is a chronic autoimmune disorder that causes inflammation of various parts of the body.
- B. Lupus is a normal part of aging that affects only women.
- C. Lupus causes an increased concentration of uric acid that leads to tophi.
- D. Lupus is characterized by multiple draining sinus tracts and metastatic lesions.

Exercise 7-35: *Fill-in*
The nurse further explains that lupus is classified into three categories, which are:

1. _____
2. _____
3. _____

Answers to this chapter begin on page 255.

Exercise 7-36: *Fill-in*

Based upon Roberta's assessment, what category of lupus is she experiencing and why?

_____

_____

Exercise 7-37: *Select all that apply*

The primary care provider has ordered a number of diagnostic tests to help confirm the diagnosis of lupus; they are:

❑ Antinuclear antibody titer

❑ Anti-Smith

❑ Anti-DNA

❑ Anti-Bob

❑ Anti-Rope

Exercise 7-38: *Multiple-choice question*

Which of these tests is the specific diagnostic marker for lupus?

A. Anti-Bob

B. Antinuclear antibody titer

C. Anti-DNA

D. Anti-Rope

Exercise 7-39: *Multiple-choice question*

Which of these tests is found only in lupus?

A. Anti-DNA

B. Anti-Smith

C. Anti-Bob

D. Anti-Rope

 eResource 7-23: To learn more about the diagnostic workup for Roberta and the diagnostic criteria, refer to Medscape on your mobile device: [Pathway: Medscape → enter "lupus" into the search field → select "Systemic Lupus Erythematosus (SLE)" → select "Workup" and review content under "Approach" and "Diagnostic Criteria for SLE"]

Exercise 7-40: *Multiple-choice question*

Roberta is distressed over the diagnosis of lupus and has more questions about how she should take care of herself and if she is contagious to others. What is the priority nursing diagnosis for Roberta?

A. Knowledge deficit

B. Chronic pain

C. Risk for altered tissue perfusion

D. Risk for infection

Answers to this chapter begin on page 255.

Exercise 7-41: *Select all that apply*

What type of teaching is provided to Roberta who has the diagnosis of lupus?

- ❏ Use sunscreen when exposed to sunlight
- ❏ Use steroid creams for skin rash
- ❏ Report signs/symptoms of infection
- ❏ Harsh hair treatments acceptable

The primary care provider (PCP) has prescribed prednisone for Roberta to help improve her symptoms.

Exercise 7-42: *Select all that apply*

The nurse should teach Roberta about what side effects of prednisone?

- ❏ Weight gain
- ❏ Loss of appetite
- ❏ Moon face
- ❏ Elevated blood glucose
- ❏ Buffalo hump
- ❏ Hair loss

eResource 7-24: To reinforce your understanding of the side effects of prednisone, refer to the following resources on your mobile device:
- ▦ Epocrates: [Pathway: Epocrates → enter "Prednisone" into the search field → scroll down to review "Adverse Reactions" and "Safety and Monitoring"]
- ▦ Skyscape's RxDrugs [Pathway: RxDrugs → enter "Prednisone" into the search field → scroll down to "warnings/precautions" and review information]
- ▦ Medscape: [Pathway: Medscape → enter "Prednisone" into the search field → select "Adverse Effects" and review information]

Answers to this chapter begin on page 255.

Answers

Exercise 7-1: *Fill-in*

The nurse suspects a possible diagnosis of: **human immunodeficiency virus (HIV) and acquired immunodeficiency syndrome (AIDS).**

Exercise 7-2: *Fill-in*

What is the significance of the CD4+ count? **It measures the number of T-helper cells affected by HIV. It predicts the HIV disease progression and also measures the effectiveness of medications against HIV.**

What is the significance of the Western blot test? **A positive Western blot test confirms an HIV infection; it also confirms a positive ELISA test. The Western blot test is more precise than the ELISA and it detects the presence of antibodies to specific antigens.**

What is the significance of an ELISA? **It is the most common and least expensive test used to diagnose HIV infection. It is used as a screening tool for AIDS. It uses an enzyme linked to an antibody or antigen as a marker for detecting a specified protein.**

Exercise 7-3: *Multiple-choice question*

What is the accepted range for the CD4+ count?
  A. 100 to 5,000 cells/mm^3—NO
  B. 500 to 1,000 cells/mm^3—YES
  C. 300 to 5,000 cells/mm^3—NO
  D. 800 to 1,000 cells/mm^3—NO

Exercise 7-4: *Multiple-choice question*

The nurse knows that CD4+ lymphocytes are also called:
  A. R-cells—NO, this is not the name.
  B. D-cells—NO, this is not the name.
  C. T-cells—YES
  D. J-cells—NO, this is not the name.

Exercise 7-5: *Fill-in*

What is the function of CD4+ lymphocytes? **CD4+ lymphocytes or T-cells attack foreign substances in the body such as bacteria, viruses, and tissues.**

Exercise 7-6: *Fill-in*

How does the primary care provider explain the differences between HIV and AIDS to Eva?

HIV is called the human immunodeficiency virus. It is a retrovirus that is transmitted by blood and body fluids. This virus targets T-cells. Individuals with HIV do not always have AIDS.

AIDS is called the acquired immunodeficiency syndrome. It occurs when the CD4+ count falls below 200 cells/mm³. At this level, the immune system cannot protect a person from AIDS infections and/or illnesses. AIDS is the end stage of HIV infection. Individuals with AIDS have the HIV infection.

Exercise 7-7: *Fill-in*

What two risk factors predisposed Eva to HIV/AIDS?

1. **IV drug use**
2. **Unprotected sex**

Exercise 7-8: *Fill-in*

What signs and symptoms did Eva present that gave the suspicion of HIV/AIDS?

1. **Fever**
2. **Diarrhea**
3. **Nausea**
4. **Vomiting**
5. **Fatigue**
6. **Night sweats**
7. **Thrush**

Exercise 7-9: *Matching*

Match the stage of HIV in Column A with its definition in Column B.

Column A		Column B
A. Stage 1: Primary HIV infection	**B**	Individuals are free from symptoms
B. Stage 2: Asymptomatic HIV	**A**	Experience flu-like symptoms; last a few weeks
C. Stage 3: AIDS	**C**	Diagnosed as having AIDS; cannot return to stage of HIV

Exercise 7-10: *Fill-in*

What stage of infection is Eva experiencing? **Stage 3: AIDS**

Exercise 7-11: *Calculation*

Calculate how many mL of Neupogen will be given subcutaneously. The vial is labeled 300 mcg/mL.

$$\frac{300 \text{ mcg}}{1} \times \frac{1 \text{ mL}}{300 \text{ mcg}} = 1 \text{ mL}$$

Exercise 7-12: *Calculation*

Calculate how many mL of Epogen will be given subcutaneously to Eva who weighs 120 pounds. The vial is labeled 4000 units/mL.

100 units	mL	1 kg	120 lb	12 = 1 × 1	= 12	= 1 mL
kg	4,000 units	2.2 lb		4 × 2.2	8.8	

Exercise 7-13: *Calculation*

Calculate how many mL/hr to set the IV pump to infuse vancomycin 500 mg. It is supplied as a 1-g vial to be reconstituted with 10 mL normal saline solution and further diluted in 100 mL D5W to infuse over 60 minutes.

500 mg	10 mL	1 g	50 × 1	= 50 = 5 mL
	1g	1,000 mg	10	10

105 mL	60 min	= 105 = 105 mL/hr
60 min	1 hr	1

Exercise 7-14: *Select all that apply*

What teaching(s) by the nurse will benefit Eva once she is discharged home?

☒ **Complying with antiretroviral medications**

☒ **Referral to AIDS support groups**

☒ **Encourage use of coping mechanisms**

☒ **Alternate activity with rest periods**

☒ **Maintain a well-balanced diet**

☒ **Follow-up with CD4+ count**

❑ Reporting signs and symptoms of infection not needed

Exercise 7-15: *Fill-in*

Why will the primary care provider order another CD4+ count?

At the first diagnosis of HIV, the first CD4+ count is a baseline measurement. A repeat CD4+ count allows the health care provider to compare measurements and to see if the anti-HIV medications are helping to fight the virus.

Exercise 7-16: *Select all that apply*

Based upon Eva's diagnosis and assessment findings, what nursing diagnoses are pertinent in her care?

☒ **Risk for infection**

❑ Imbalanced nutrition: more than body requirements

☒ **Ineffective coping**

☒ **Fatigue/activity intolerance**

☒ **Imbalanced nutrition: less than body requirements**

Exercise 7-17: *Fill-in*

What is rheumatoid arthritis? **Rheumatoid arthritis is a chronic systemic disease that affects various joints in the body and causes swelling, pain, stiffness, and inflammation.**

Exercise 7-18: *Fill-in*

The hallmark symptom in rheumatoid arthritis is **pain.**

Exercise 7-19: *Select all that apply*

What are risk factors for rheumatoid arthritis?

☒ **Female gender**

☒ **Age 30 to 50 years**

☒ **Family history**

☒ **Smoking**

❑ Diet high in protein

Exercise 7-20: *Fill-in*

What do these tests tell us as it relates to rheumatoid arthritis?

1. RF antibody **The diagnostic level for rheumatoid arthritis is 1:40 to 1:60; normal level is 1:20 or less. If the titer is high, it correlates with the severity of the disease.**
2. ESR **is associated with inflammation or infection in the body. Levels are: 20 to 40 mm/hr = mild inflammation; 40 to 70 mm/hr = moderate inflammation; and 70 to 150 mm/hr = severe inflammation.**
3. ANA titer **A positive titer is associated with rheumatoid arthritis. A normal titer is negative at 1:20 dilution.**
4. WBC count **will be elevated due to the inflammatory response.**

Exercise 7-21: *Matching*

Match the diagnostic imaging test in Column A to its procedure in Column B.

Column A		Column B
A. Dual energy x-ray absorptiometry	**C**	Detects bone erosions in hands in rheumatoid arthritis
B. Ultrasound	**B**	Monitors inflammatory activity
C. Magnetic resonance imaging	**A**	Detects early bone loss in rheumatoid arthritis

Exercise 7-22: *Multiple-choice question*

What is the priority nursing diagnosis for Mabel based upon the nurse's assessment?

A. Fatigue—NO, although this may be an issue, it is not the priority.

B. Pain—YES, this is the priority.

C. Disturbed body image—NO, although this may be an issue, it is not the priority.

D. Impaired physical mobility—NO

Exercise 7-23: *Fill-in*

Name three side effects of Plaquenil.

1. **Headache**
2. **Nausea**
3. **Rash**

Exercise 7-24: *Fill-in*

Name three side effects of Humira.

1. **Fever**
2. **Vomiting**
3. **Bleeding**

Exercise 7-25: *Multiple-choice question*

Mabel needs further discharge teaching when she says:

A. "I am to pace my activities by resting for 5 to 10 minutes."—NO, she should rest.

B. "I am to take my prescribed medications as directed."—NO, she should take her medication.

C. "I can take a hot shower or bath to reduce the need for pain medication."—NO, heat will help the pain.

D. **"I don't have to watch my weight with rheumatoid arthritis."—YES, weight will add to the burden of the joints.**

Exercise 7-26 *Fill-in*

Georgia's signs and symptoms are indicative of **osteoarthritis.**

Exercise 7-27: *Fill-in*

What differentiates this disease process from rheumatoid arthritis?

It is a noninflammatory nonsystemic disease that is a progressive deterioration of articular cartilage.

Exercise 7-28: *Select all that apply*

Identify some risk factors for osteoarthritis.

☒ **Age**

☒ **Decreased muscle strength**

☒ **Obesity**

☒ **Genetic predisposition**

❑ Hypertension

Exercise 7-29: *Select all that apply*

The nurse has assessed nodules on Georgia's hands. The nurse knows that the following type(s) of nodes are easily recognizable signs of osteoarthritis:

☒ **Heberden's nodes**

❑ Wilmer's nodes

☒ **Bouchard's nodes**

❑ Lymph nodes

Exercise 7-30: *Select all that apply*
What alternative methods can be utilized to reduce pain and discomfort of the joints?

☒ **Moist heat to joints**

☒ **Massage of joints**

☒ **Adequate rest after activities**

☒ **Gentle range-of-motion exercises**

☒ **Proper body mechanics**

Exercise 7-31: *Select all that apply*
Georgia complained of pain and a decrease in her activities due to the osteoarthritis. Based on this assessment, what are the two top nursing diagnoses for Georgia?

☒ **Pain—YES**

☒ **Activity intolerance—YES**

❑ Disturbed body image—NO, this is not the priority, although it may be an issue.

❑ Impaired skin integrity—NO, this is not the priority, although it may be an issue.

Exercise 7-32: *Fill-in*
Identify which characteristics are indicative of osteoarthritis or rheumatoid arthritis:
Heberden's nodes **Osteoarthritis**
Progressive deterioration of articular cartilage **Osteoarthritis**
Pain occurs with activity **Osteoarthritis**
Autoimmune response **Rheumatoid arthritis**
Systemic response **Rheumatoid arthritis**

Exercise 7-33: *Select all that apply*
What sign and symptoms in Roberta's assessment indicates a diagnosis of systemic lupus erythematosus (SLE)?

☒ **Butterfly rash**

☒ **Weakness**

☒ **Malaise**

☒ **Low-grade fever**

☒ **Joint inflammation**

❑ Tonsillectomy

Exercise 7-34: *Multiple-choice question*
Roberta does not understand lupus and asks the nurse what caused her to have this disease. The nurse explains to her that:

A. **Lupus is a chronic autoimmune disorder that causes inflammation of various parts of the body.—YES, this is a good explanation.**

B. Lupus is a normal part of aging that affects only women.—NO, this is not true.

C. Lupus causes an increased concentration of uric acid that leads to tophi.—NO, this is not true.

D. Lupus is characterized by multiple draining sinus tracts and metastatic lesions.—NO, this is not true.

Exercise 7-35: *Fill-in*
The nurse further explains that lupus is classified into three categories, which are:
1. **Discoid**
2. **Systemic**
3. **Drug-induced**

Exercise 7-36: *Fill-in*
Based upon Roberta's assessment, what category of lupus is she experiencing and why.
She is exhibiting signs of discoid and systemic lupus. She has the classic butterfly rash on the face/cheek area, which affects the skin, and her sight and joints are being affected, which is systemic.

Exercise 7-37: *Select all that apply*
The primary care provider has ordered a number of diagnostic tests to help confirm the diagnosis of lupus, which are:
☒ **Antinuclear antibody titer**
☒ **Anti-Smith**
☒ **Anti-DNA**
❑ Anti-Bob
❑ Anti-Rope

Exercise 7-38: *Multiple-choice question*
Which of these tests is the specific diagnostic marker for lupus?
A. Anti-Bob—NO, this is not specific for SLE.
B. Antinuclear antibody titer—YES
C. Anti-DNA—NO, this is not specific for SLE.
D. Anti-Rope—NO, this is not specific for SLE.

Exercise 7-39: *Multiple-choice question*
Which of these tests is found only in lupus?
A. Anti-DNA—NO, this is not specific for SLE.
B. Anti-Smith—YES
C. Anti-Bob—NO, this is not specific for SLE.
D. Anti-Rope—NO, this is not specific for SLE.

Exercise 7-40: *Multiple-choice question*

Roberta is distressed over the diagnosis of lupus and has more questions about how she should take care of herself and if she is contagious to others. What is the priority nursing diagnosis for Roberta?

 A. Knowledge deficit—YES, this is the most pressing need for the patient.
 B. Chronic pain—NO, this is not the priority right now.
 C. Risk for altered tissue perfusion—NO, this is not the priority right now.
 D. Risk for infection—NO, this is not the priority right now.

Exercise 7-41: *Select all that apply*

What type of teaching is provided to Roberta who has the diagnosis of lupus?

☒ **Use sunscreen when exposed to sunlight**

☒ **Use steroid creams for skin rash**

☒ **Report signs/symptoms of infection**

❑ Harsh hair treatments acceptable

Exercise 7-42: *Select all that apply*

The nurse should teach Roberta about what side effects of prednisone?

☒ **Weight gain**

❑ Loss of appetite

☒ **Moon face**

☒ **Elevated blood glucose**

☒ **Buffalo hump**

❑ Hair loss

8

Nursing Care of the Patient With Hematological Disease

Karen K. Gittings

Unfolding Case Study #43 ▦ Whitney

Whitney is a 25-year-old mother of three young children. At her annual gyneco-logical appointment, Whitney reports that she always feels so tired and even weak at times. The nurse observes that Whitney has a pale color and is wearing a sweat-shirt on a warm summer day. Her vital signs are within normal range except for her pulse, which is slightly tachycardic at 102 beats/min. The nurse suspects that Whitney is exhibiting clinical manifestations of anemia.

Exercise 8-1: *Fill-in*

Identify the three classifications of anemia based on physiological cause with a brief explanation of each:

1. _____
2. _____
3. _____

Exercise 8-2: *Fill-in*

For each classification of anemia, identify two examples that would fall under this category/classification:

Classification #1 _____

    a. _____

    b. _____

Classification #2 _____

    a. _____

    b. _____

Classification #3 _____

    a. _____

    b. _____

Answers to this chapter begin on page 273.

eResource 8-1: Refer to Medscape to reinforce your understanding of anemia: [Pathway: Medscape → enter "anemia" into the search field → select "anemia" → review content in "overview." Be sure to review content under "etiology"]

While being seen by the primary care provider (PCP), Whitney also mentions that she has heavy menstrual cycles every month. The PCP informs her that based on her history of heavy menstrual cycles and her current signs and symptoms, she likely has iron-deficiency anemia. To confirm the diagnosis, the PCP orders a complete blood count (CBC) with red blood cell (RBC) indices and ferritin level. Whitney is advised to start taking a multivitamin with iron and is instructed to follow-up in the office in 2 weeks.

Exercise 8-3: *Select all that apply*

Identify other clinical manifestations of iron-deficiency anemia.

❑ Beefy, red, sore tongue

❑ Pica

❑ Paresthesia

❑ Cold intolerance

❑ Dyspnea

 eResource 8-2: To reinforce your understanding of the clinical manifestations of anemia, refer to:
- ▦ Medscape on your mobile device: [Pathway: Medscape → enter "anemia" into the search field → select "anemia" → select "Clinical Presentation" and review content]
- ▦ View *Anemia 1: Overview & Iron Deficiency Anemia:* http://youtu.be/45v4R1S-2Hw

Exercise 8-4: *Matching*

Match the RBC indices in Column A with their description in Column B.

Column A	Column B
A. Mean corpuscular volume (MCV)	_____ Average mass of hemoglobin per red blood cell; normal value is 28 to 33 pg
B. Mean corpuscular hemoglobin (MCH)	_____ Measure of concentration of hemoglobin in a given volume of packed red blood cells; normal value is 33% to 35%
C. Mean corpuscular hemoglobin concentration (MCHC)	_____ Measure of average red blood cell size; normal value is 84 to 96 fL

Answers to this chapter begin on page 273.

Exercise 8-5: *True or false*
Identify whether the following statements about diagnostic findings associated with iron-deficiency anemia are true or false:

_____ 1. A low ferritin level, which is seen in iron-deficiency anemia, indicates that iron levels are depleted.

_____ 2. Total RBCs, hemoglobin (Hgb), and hematocrit (Hct) are decreased with iron-deficiency anemia.

_____ 3. The RBC indices (MCV, MCH, and MCHC) are high with iron-deficiency anemia.

_____ 4. A low serum iron level and low total iron-binding capacity (TIBC) are indicative of iron-deficiency anemia.

 eResource 8-3: For more information about iron-deficiency anemia, refer to Medscape on your mobile device: [Pathway: Medscape → enter "anemia" into the search field → select "anemia" → select "Differential Diagnoses" → select "Iron Deficiency Anemia" and review content]

Exercise 8-6: *Multiple-choice question*
When describing the red blood cell morphology associated with iron-deficiency anemia, the nurse tells her patient that cells should be:

A. Macrocytic and normochromic

B. Normocytic and normochromic

C. Macrocytic and hypochromic

D. Microcytic and hypochromic

Whitney's lab results all support the diagnosis of iron-deficiency anemia. The nurse explains that iron-deficiency anemia is the most common type of anemia and in premenopausal women, it is often associated with menorrhagia and/or inadequate iron in the diet.

 eResource 8-4: For more information about the epidemiology of iron-deficiency anemia, refer to Medscape on your mobile device: [Pathway: Medscape → enter "Iron Deficiency Anemia" into the search field → under "Overview" select "Epidemiology" and review content]

Whitney's PCP has decided to prescribe a prescription-strength iron supplement, ferrous sulfate 324 mg orally twice a day. Since dietary sources are also important, the nurse discusses foods high in iron.

Exercise 8-7: *Select all that apply*
Identify food sources high in iron:

❑ Citrus fruits

❑ Organ meats

❑ Leafy, green vegetables

❑ Pinto beans

❑ Milk

Answers to this chapter begin on page 273.

eResource 8-5: To learn more about dietary measures to treat iron-deficiency anemia, refer to the National Institutes of Health's publication *How Is Anemia Treated?* http://goo.gl/7x8Cf

Exercise 8-8: *Fill-in*

Identify three common side effects associated with iron supplements:

1. _____

2. _____

3. _____

Exercise 8-9: *Select all that apply*

Identify important teaching points for the patient who is newly prescribed an iron supplement:

❏ Take iron on an empty stomach as tolerated to increase absorption

❏ Increase intake of vitamin C food sources to increase iron absorption

❏ Take an antacid or dairy product with the iron supplement to enhance absorption

❏ Avoid a diet high in fiber, which can interfere with iron absorption

❏ If a liquid iron supplement is prescribed, use a straw or a spoon to place the iron at the back of the mouth to prevent staining

 eResource 8-6: To learn more about ferrous sulfate, consult the following resources on your mobile device:

▦ Medscape: [Pathway: Medscape → enter "ferrous sulfate" into the search field → review content]

▦ Skyscape's RxDrugs: [Pathway: RxDrugs → enter "ferrous sulfate" into the search field → review content]

▦ Epocrates: [Pathway: Epocrates → enter "ferrous sulfate" into the search field → review content]

Exercise 8-10: *Fill-in*

Identify three food sources high in vitamin C:

1. _____

2. _____

3. _____

After discussing diet and iron supplementation with Whitney, the nurse asks if she has any further questions or concerns. Whitney states that she is primarily having difficulty with feeling so tired all the time, so she questions when she will start feeling better and if there is anything else she can do in the meantime.

Exercise 8-11: *Fill-in*

Identify three nursing diagnoses for the patient with iron-deficiency anemia:

1. _____

2. _____

3. _____

Exercise 8-12: *Multiple-choice question*

When discussing interventions for managing her fatigue, the nurse determines that Whitney understands the information when she states:

    A. "I will try to minimize all physical activity until I start to feel better."

    B. "I will try to get at least 12 hours of sleep a night."

    C. "I need to rest at least once per hour."

    D. "I need to establish priorities and find a balance between activity and rest."

e   **eResource 8-7:** For supplemental information to assist in development of a nursing care plan for Whitney to help address her fatigue, refer to Nursing Care Plan and Diagnosis: http://goo.gl/8xccA

Exercise 8-13: *Short answer*

Briefly explain how long it will take to correct Whitney's iron-deficiency anemia and when she can expect to start feeling better.

_____

_____

_____

_____

Unfolding Case Study #44   Dale

Dale is a 68-year-old male who was originally admitted to a medical unit with the diagnosis of urinary tract infection. He was a resident of a long-term care facility. His past medical history includes hypertension, myocardial infarction, congestive heart failure, diabetes, benign prostatic hypertrophy, and dementia. He is currently in the medical intensive care unit with urosepsis. Over the past 3 days, there has been a steady decline in Dale's platelet count. Today, the nurse notes that Dale has blood oozing from his intravenous sites and old venipuncture sites. He also has blood in his urine and a small amount of blood is draining from his nasogastric tube. The primary care provider (PCP) suspects that Dale is developing disseminated intravascular coagulation (DIC).

Exercise 8-14: *Select all that apply*

Disseminated intravascular coagulation (DIC) is not a disease, but a sign of another underlying condition. Identify conditions that may trigger the onset of DIC:

❑ Sepsis

❑ Shock

❑ Trauma

❑ Myocardial infarction

❑ Allergic reactions

❑ Abruptio placentae

❑ Status asthmaticus

Exercise 8-15: *Short answer*

In DIC, both clotting and bleeding occur in the body. Briefly explain the pathophysiology behind this occurrence.

_____

_____

_____

_____

e **eResource 8-8:** To learn more about the pathophysiology of DIC, consult:
- Medscape on your mobile device Medscape: [Pathway: Medscape → enter "DIC" into the search field → select "Pathophysiology" and review content]
- View the iMedicalSchool video, *Disseminated Intravascular Coagulation (DIC)*: http://youtu.be/3gBdiXpwHAE

Exercise 8-16: *True or false*

Identify whether the following statements about DIC are true or false:

_____ 1. In DIC, organ function declines as a result of ischemia caused by microthrombi or, to a lesser extent, bleeding.

_____ 2. The fibrinolytic system releases fibrin degradation products to assist with coagulation.

_____ 3. Successfully treating DIC also involves treating the underlying condition that served as the initial trigger.

Exercise 8-17: *Select all that apply*

Identify clinical manifestations that may occur related to microthrombi or bleeding associated with DIC:

❑ Petechiae

❑ Increased urine output

❑ Altered level of consciousness

Answers to this chapter begin on page 273.

❑ Hematemesis

❑ Bradycardia

❑ Cyanosis in extremities

❑ Hypoxia

 eResource 8-9: To learn more about the clinical manifestations of DIC, consult:

■ Epocrates Online: [Pathway: → http://online.epocrates.com → select the "diseases" tab → enter "DIC" into the search field → select "disseminated intravascular coagulation (DIC)" and review "Key Highlights" and "Physical Exam"]

■ Medscape on your mobile device: [Pathway: Medscape → enter "DIC" into the search field → select "Clinical Presentation" and review content]

Dale's PCP orders multiple laboratory tests to confirm his diagnosis of DIC. Since he suspects that the DIC has been triggered by Dale's urosepsis, an infectious disease specialist has also been consulted to evaluate and confirm that Dale is receiving the most effective antibiotics for fighting the bacterial infection.

Exercise 8-18: *Matching*

Match the laboratory test in Column A with its normal range and the function it is evaluating in Column B.

Column A	Column B
A. Platelet count	_____ 0 to 250 ng/mL; evaluates local fibrinolysis
B. Prothrombin time (PT)	_____ 23 to 35 seconds; evaluates intrinsic pathway
C. Partial thromboplastin time (aPTT)	_____ 0 to 5 mcg/mL; evaluates fibrinolysis
D. Fibrinogen	_____ 150,000 to 450,000/mm³; evaluates number of platelets
E. D-dimer	_____ 11 to 12.5 seconds; evaluates extrinsic pathway
F. Fibrin degradation products (FDPs)	_____ 170 to 340 mg/dL; evaluates amount available for coagulation

 eResource 8-10: To reinforce your understanding of normal blood values, refer to the University of Minnesota's medical student website, *Normal Lab Values*: http://goo.gl/sTM1A

Exercise 8-19: *Fill-in*

Identify whether the following laboratory tests would be expected to increase or decrease in the patient with DIC:

1. Platelet count   _____

2. Prothrombin time (PT)   _____

3. Partial thromboplastin time (aPTT)   _____

4. Fibrinogen   _____

5. D-dimer   _____

6. Fibrin degradation products (FDPs)   _____

 eResource 8-11: To reinforce your understanding of lab results that indicate DIC, refer to Medscape on your mobile device: [Pathway: Medscape → enter "DIC" into the search field → select "Workup" → select "Laboratory Studies" and review content]

Dale's laboratory results support the diagnosis of DIC. The infectious disease specialist has changed some of Dale's antibiotics to optimize the treatment of his urosepsis. Dale is already being aggressively treated with intravenous fluids and oxygen to maintain tissue perfusion and oxygenation. A complete blood count (CBC), basic metabolic panel (BMP), and coagulation profile are ordered every 12 hours. Dale is monitored closely for signs of increased bleeding and deterioration.

Exercise 8-20: *Matching*

Match the blood product in Column A with its indication for use in Column B.

Column A	Column B
A. Platelets	_____ Increases red blood cell mass; for symptomatic anemia
B. Fresh-frozen plasma	_____ For bleeding due to severe decrease in platelets
C. Cryoprecipitate	_____ Replaces coagulation factor deficiencies in patients who are bleeding
D. Packed red blood cells	_____ Replaces fibrinogen and factors V and VII

 eResource 8-12: To learn more about blood products, refer to the Merck Manual: [Pathway: www.merckmanuals.com → select "Merck Manual of Diagnosis and Therapy" → enter "Blood Products" into the search field → select "Blood Products" → scroll down to review content]

Exercise 8-21: *Short answer*
Briefly explain the controversial use of heparin in treating DIC.

_____

_____

_____

_____

_____

eResource 8-13: To reinforce your understanding:
- Review the iMedical School video: *Disseminated Intravascular Coagulation (DIC)*: http://youtu.be/3gBdiXpwHAE
- View, *DIC* video lecture by Dr. Sue Gamel-McCormick: http://youtu.be/87uBWZmZGWk

Exercise 8-22: *Select all that apply*
Identify nursing interventions that will prevent or minimize bleeding associated with DIC:

❑ Avoid intramuscular (IM) injections
❑ Use high pressure with any suctioning
❑ Avoid dislodging any clots
❑ Avoid rectal medications or probes
❑ Use nonsteroidal anti-inflammatory drugs instead of aspirin
❑ Use soft, sponge-tipped mouth swabs
❑ Avoid lemon-glycerine swabs

eResource 8-14: For additional resources to develop a nursing care plan for Dale, consult eNurse Care Plans: http://goo.gl/4P3fg

Answers

Exercise 8-1: *Fill-in*

Identify the three classifications of anemia based on physiological cause with a brief explanation of each:

1. **Hypoproliferative—defect in production of red blood cells**
2. **Hemolytic—destruction of red blood cells**
3. **Blood loss—bleeding**

Exercise 8-2: *Fill-in*

For each classification of anemia, identify two examples that would fall under this category/classification:

Classification #1 **Hypoproliferative**

a. **Iron deficiency**
b. **Vitamin B$_{12}$ deficiency**
c. **Folate deficiency**
d. **Decreased production related to renal dysfunction**

Classification #2 **Hemolytic**

a. **Sickle cell anemia**
b. **Autoimmune anemia**
c. **Heart valve–related anemia**
d. **Hypersplenism**

Classification #3 **Bleeding**

a. **Bleeding from gastrointestinal tract**
b. **Bleeding from genitourinary tract**
c. **Trauma**

Exercise 8-3: *Select all that apply*

Identify other clinical manifestations of iron-deficiency anemia:

☐ Beefy, red, sore tongue—NO, this is found with vitamin B$_{12}$ deficiencies.

☒ **Pica—YES, this is a craving of nonfood products, such as ice, starch, or dirt.**

☐ Paresthesia—NO, this is found with vitamin B$_{12}$ deficiencies.

☒ **Cold intolerance—YES**

☒ **Dyspnea—YES, with anemia there is less hemoglobin to transport oxygen.**

Exercise 8-4: *Matching*
Match the red blood cell (RBC) indices in Column A with its description in Column B.

Column A		Column B
A. MCV	**B**	Average mass of hemoglobin per red blood cell; normal value is 28 to 33 pg
B. MCH	**C**	Measure of concentration of hemoglobin in a given volume of packed red blood cells; normal value is 33% to 35%
C. MCHC	**A**	Measure of average red blood cell size; normal value is 84 to 96 fL

Exercise 8-5: *True or false*
Identify whether the following statements about diagnostic findings associated with iron-deficiency anemia are true or false:

True 1. A low ferritin level, which is seen in iron-deficiency anemia, indicates that iron levels are depleted.

True 2. Total red blood cells (RBCs), hemoglobin (Hgb), and hematocrit (Hct) are decreased with iron-deficiency anemia.

False 3. The RBC indices (MCV, MCH, and MCHC) are high with iron-deficiency anemia.

False 4. A low serum iron level and low total iron-binding capacity (TIBC) are indicative of iron-deficiency anemia.

Exercise 8-6: *Multiple-choice question*
When describing the red blood cell morphology associated with iron-deficiency anemia, the nurse tells her patient that cells should be:

A. Macrocytic and normochromic—NO, this is associated with folic acid or vitamin B_{12} deficiency.

B. Normocytic and normochromic—NO, this is seen in normal cells.

C. Macrocytic and hypochromic—NO

D. Microcytic and hypochromic—YES, this is associated with iron-deficiency anemia.

Exercise 8-7: *Select all that apply*
Identify food sources high in iron:

❑ Citrus fruits—NO

☒ **Organ meats—YES, such as beef, calf, or chicken liver.**

☒ **Leafy, green vegetables—YES, such as broccoli, lettuce, or collard greens.**

☒ **Pinto beans—YES**

❑ Milk—NO

Exercise 8-8: *Fill-in*

Identify three common side effects associated with iron supplements:

1. **Constipation**
2. **Nausea/vomiting**
3. **Cramping**
4. **Epigastric pain**
5. **Dark stools**

Exercise 8-9: *Select all that apply*

Identify important teaching points for the patient who is newly prescribed an iron supplement:

☒ **Take iron on an empty stomach as tolerated to increase absorption—YES, this is recommended if the patient can tolerate it.**

☒ **Increase intake of vitamin C food sources to increase iron absorption—YES**

❑ Take an antacid or dairy product with the iron supplement to enhance absorption—NO, this will greatly diminish iron absorption.

❑ Avoid a diet high in fiber, which can interfere with iron absorption—NO, a high-fiber diet is recommended to prevent constipation.

☒ **If a liquid iron supplement is prescribed, use a straw or a spoon to place the iron at the back of the mouth to prevent staining—YES**

Exercise 8-10: *Fill-in*

Identify three food sources high in vitamin C:

1. **Citrus fruit and juices**
2. **Broccoli**
3. **Cantaloupe**
4. **Strawberries**
5. **Tomatoes**

Exercise 8-11: *Fill-in*

Identify three nursing diagnoses for the patient with iron-deficiency anemia:

1. **Fatigue related to diminished oxygen-carrying capacity of the blood**
2. **Activity intolerance related to diminished oxygen-carrying capacity of the blood**
3. **Anxiety related to new diagnosis and treatment regimen**
4. **Altered nutrition, less than body requirements, related to inadequate intake of iron**
5. **Alteration in tissue perfusion related to decreased hemoglobin and hematocrit**

Exercise 8-12: *Multiple-choice question*
When discussing interventions for managing her fatigue, the nurse determines that Whitney understands the information when she states:
A. "I will try to minimize all physical activity until I start to feel better."—NO
B. "I will try to get at least 12 hours of sleep a night."—NO
C. "I need to rest at least once per hour."—NO
D. "I need to establish priorities and find a balance between activity and rest."
 —YES, this is the best plan until the fatigue lessens as the anemia improves.

Exercise 8-13: *Short answer*
Briefly explain how long it will take to correct Whitney's iron-deficiency anemia and when she can expect to start feeling better.
With treatment, hemoglobin levels will start increasing in 2 to 3 weeks, and the anemia can be corrected in only a few months. As the hemoglobin increases and the anemia improves, the patient will begin seeing an improvement in symptoms. It is important, though, for the patient to continue treatment despite feeling better because it may take 6 to 12 months to replenish iron stores.

Exercise 8-14: *Select all that apply*
Disseminated intravascular coagulation (DIC) is not a disease, but a sign of another underlying condition. Identify conditions that may trigger the onset of DIC:
☒ **Sepsis—YES**
☒ **Shock—YES**
☒ **Trauma—YES**
❑ Myocardial infarction—NO, this is not a known trigger.
☒ **Allergic reactions—YES**
☒ **Abruptio placentae—YES**
❑ Status asthmaticus—NO, this is not a known trigger.

Exercise 8-15: *Short answer*
In DIC, both clotting and bleeding occur in the body. Briefly explain the pathophysiology behind this occurrence.
DIC occurs when the inflammation caused by an underlying disease process, such as sepsis, initiates the coagulation cascade, but the anticoagulant pathways and fibrinolytic system are not functioning properly. Numerous tiny clots form, leading to consumption of platelets and clotting factors. Eventually, as coagulation fails, bleeding occurs.

Exercise 8-16: *True or false*

Identify whether the following statements about DIC are true or false:

True   1. In DIC, organ function declines as a result of ischemia caused by micro-thrombi or to a lesser extent, bleeding.

False 2. The fibrinolytic system releases fibrin degradation products to assist with coagulation.

True   3. Successfully treating DIC also involves treating the underlying condition that served as the initial trigger.

Exercise 8-17: *Select all that apply*

Identify clinical manifestations that may occur related to microthrombi or bleeding associated with DIC:

☒ **Petechiae—YES, a result of microvascular bleeding.**

❑ Increased urine output—NO, urine output would be decreased related to microthrombi or overall blood loss.

☒ **Altered level of consciousness—YES, may be related to microthrombi or bleeding in the brain.**

☒ **Hematemesis—YES, this is a result of bleeding in the gastrointestinal tract.**

❑ Bradycardia—NO, tachycardia would occur, especially with blood loss.

☒ **Cyanosis in extremities—YES, a result of microthrombi.**

☒ **Hypoxia—YES, if thrombi develop in the lungs.**

Exercise 8-18: *Matching*

Match the laboratory test in Column A with its normal range and the function it is evaluating in Column B.

Column A		Column B
A. Platelet count	**E**	0 to 250 ng/mL; evaluates local fibrinolysis
B. Prothrombin time (PT)	**C**	23 to 35 seconds; evaluates intrinsic pathway
C. Partial thromboplastin time (aPTT)	**F**	0 to 5 mcg/mL; evaluates fibrinolysis
D. Fibrinogen	**A**	150,000 to 450,000/mm³; evaluates number of platelets
E. D-dimer	**B**	11 to 12.5 seconds; evaluates extrinsic pathway
F. Fibrin degradation products (FDPs)	**D**	170 to 340 mg/dL; evaluates amount available for coagulation

Exercise 8-19: *Fill-in*

Identify whether the following laboratory tests would be expected to increase or decrease in the patient with DIC:

1. Platelet count   **Decrease**
2. Prothrombin time (PT)   **Increase**
3. Partial thromboplastin time (aPTT)   **Increase**
4. Fibrinogen   **Decrease**
5. D-dimer   **Increase**
6. Fibrin degradation products (FDPs)   **Increase**

Exercise 8-20: *Matching*

Match the blood product in Column A with its indication for use in Column B.

Column A		Column B
A. Platelets	**D**	Increases red blood cell mass; for symptomatic anemia
B. Fresh-frozen plasma	**A**	For bleeding due to severe decrease in platelets
C. Cryoprecipitate	**B**	Replaces coagulation factor deficiencies in patients who are bleeding
D. Packed red blood cells	**C**	Replaces fibrinogen and factors V and VII

Exercise 8-21: *Short answer*

Briefly explain the controversial use of heparin in treating DIC.

Although heparin is contraindicated with uncontrolled bleeding, it has been used with DIC to interrupt the process of thrombosis. By inhibiting microthrombi, organ perfusion can resume. Heparin was traditionally used when thrombosis predominated or when blood replacement therapy was unsuccessful in halting bleeding, but today it may be used even with less severe forms of DIC.

Exercise 8-22: *Select all that apply*

Identify nursing interventions that will prevent or minimize bleeding associated with DIC:

☒ **Avoid intramuscular (IM) injections—YES, decreases intramuscular bleeding.**

❑ Use high pressure with any suctioning—NO, use low pressure to reduce bleeding from trauma.

☒ **Avoid dislodging any clots—YES, prevents re-bleeding at sites.**

☒ **Avoid rectal medications or probes—YES, decreases rectal bleeding.**

❑ Use nonsteroidal anti-inflammatory drugs instead of aspirin—NO, these interfere with platelet function.

☒ **Use soft, sponge-tipped mouth swabs—YES, prevents excessive trauma to mouth.**

☒ **Avoid lemon-glycerine swabs—YES, these are drying, which increases bleeding risk.**

9

Nursing Care of the Patient With Musculoskeletal Disease

Rhonda M. Brogdon

Unfolding Case Study #45 ▪ Frances

Frances is a 66-year-old patient who has come to her primary care provider (PCP) complaining of back pain when she bends. She rates her pain a 5 on a numerical scale of 0 to 10, with 10 being the highest. Frances has become more sedentary and has not been eating well since the pain has begun. She states that her dietary intake has been low and she has started to smoke cigarettes again after being cigarette free for 6 years. Frances has a medical history of estrogen therapy for hot flashes, smoker for 15 years, urinary tract infections, and a fractured right wrist. Francis has a family history of hypertension and diabetes.

Exercise 9-1: *Fill-in*
Based on Frances' signs and symptoms, the nurse suspects: _____.

Exercise 9-2: *Select all that apply*
Frances asks the nurse, "What has led to me having this condition?" The nurse explains to Frances risk factors that may lead to osteoporosis.

❑ Family history

❑ Female

❑ Age over 60

❑ Smoking history

❑ Prolonged immobility

❑ Postmenopausal estrogen deficiency

❑ Thick, lean body

e **eResource 9-1:** To supplement your understanding of the risk factors associated with osteoporosis, refer to Epocrates Online: [Pathway: http://online.epocrates.com → select the "Diseases" tab → enter "Osteoporosis" into the search field → under "Diagnosis" select "risk factors" and review content]

Answers to this chapter begin on page 287.

ⓔ **eResource 9-2:** To help Frances better understand osteoporosis, the nurse shows her the following videos:
■ *Osteoporosis-3D Medical Animation*: http://http://youtu.be/rHyeZhcoZcQ
■ MedlinePlus's *Osteoporosis*: http://goo.gl/pj1xb

Exercise 9-3: *Select all that apply*

The primary care provider has ordered laboratory tests to determine the severity of Frances' osteoporosis. What types of laboratory tests are pertinent in ruling out other musculoskeletal disorders?

❑ Serum potassium

❑ Serum calcium

❑ Vitamin D

❑ Vitamin A

❑ Phosphorus

❑ Alkaline phosphatase

ⓔ **eResource 9-3:** To learn more about the relevant laboratory tests for osteoporosis, refer to:
■ Medscape on your mobile device: [Pathway: Medscape → enter "osteoporosis" into the search field → select "workup" → select "Laboratory Studies" and review content]
■ The Merck Manual: [Pathway: www.merckmanuals.com → select "Merck Manual of Diagnosis and Therapy" → enter "osteoporosis" into the search field → select "osteoporosis" → select "Etiology" and review content]

Exercise 9-4: *Matching*

The PCP has ordered three diagnostic procedures to determine the bone changes that have occurred.

Match the term in Column A to the definition in Column B.

Column A	Column B
A. Radiographs	_____ Determines osteoporosis and assesses risk for fracture
B. Quantitative ultrasound	_____ Reveals low bone density and fractures
C. Dual energy x-ray absorptiometry	_____ Measures bone mineral density in wrist, hip, and vertebral column

ⓔ **eResource 9-4:** To supplement your teaching regarding the diagnostic procedures, refer to:
■ MedlinePlus for information re: Bone Density Test: [Pathway: www.nlm.nih.gov/medlineplus → enter "bone density test" into the search field → select "bone density mineral test" and review content]

Answers to this chapter begin on page 287.

■ American Academy of Orthopedic Surgeons (AAOS): [Pathway: http://orthoinfo.aaos.org → enter "osteoporosis" into the search field → scroll down and select "Osteoporosis Tests" and review content. (Note: There are many diagnostic procedures related to osteoporosis listed here)]

Frances asks the nurse what types of food she can eat to help increase her calcium levels.

Exercise 9-5: *Multiple-choice question*
To minimize further damage or risks of osteoporosis, the nurse would recommend which of the following foods for Frances?

A. Bread/fish
B. Chicken/oranges
C. Milk/yogurt
D. Oatmeal/rice

 eResource 9-5: For more information regarding dietary treatment, refer to:
■ Epocrates Online: [Pathway: http://online.epocrates.com → select the "diseases" tab → enter "osteoporosis" into the search field → select "Treatment" tab → review content under "Approach," focusing on "Diet and Lifestyle"]
■ The Merck Manual: [Pathway: www.merckmanuals.com → select "Merck Manual of Diagnosis and Therapy" → enter "osteoporosis" into the search field → select "osteoporosis" → select "Treatment" and review content. Be sure to review content regarding "preventing bone loss"]

Exercise 9-6: *Select all that apply*
The primary care provider has prescribed Premarin 0.625 mg daily, calcium carbonate 500 mg twice a day, vitamin D 800 IU daily, and Fosamax 10 mg daily for Frances. What side effects do these medications have in common?

❑ Headache
❑ Nausea
❑ Slow heart rate
❑ Sore eyes
❑ Vomiting
❑ Poor appetite

 eResource 9-6: To reinforce your understanding of these medications, their effects and side effects, refer to the following resources on your mobile device:
■ Epocrates: [Pathway: Epocrates → enter "Premarin" into the search field and review information. Repeat this activity with calcium carbonate, vitamin D, and Fosamax]

Answers to this chapter begin on page 287.

■ Skyscape's RxDrugs: [Pathway: RxDrugs → enter "Premarin" into the search field and review information. Repeat this activity with calcium carbonate, vitamin D, and Fosamax]

■ Medscape: [Pathway: Medscape → enter "Premarin" into the search field and review information. Repeat this activity with calcium carbonate, vitamin D, and Fosamax]

Exercise 9-7: *Select all that apply*

The nurse knows Frances' care will comprise which nursing diagnoses?

❑ Activity intolerance

❑ Imbalanced nutrition: more than body requirements

❑ Risk for falls

❑ Acute pain

Exercise 9-8: *Fill-in*

Frances is concerned about having fractures with her diagnosis of osteoporosis. The nurse explains to Frances that fractures are:

_____

_____

Exercise 9-9: *Select all that apply*

The nurse knows what interventions are important for Frances with the diagnosis of osteoporosis.

❑ Use safety equipment

❑ Educate the importance of regular, weight-bearing exercises

❑ Reinforce the need to consume dietary calcium food sources

❑ Educate on taking calcium before eating

❑ Remove throw rugs in home, ensure adequate lighting, clear walkway

e **eResource 9-7:** To reinforce patient teaching, the nurse consults Epocrates Online: [Pathway: http://online.epocrates.com → select the "diseases" tab → enter "osteoporosis" into the search field → select "treatment" tab → select "prevention" and review content related to primary and secondary prevention]

Unfolding Case Study #46 ■ Vera

Vera is a 76-year-old patient with a history of osteoporosis and has been a cigarette smoker for 25 years. She has been accompanied by her son to the emergency department (ED). Her son found her on the floor in the kitchen, and she was complaining of pain in her right hip. Vera rated her pain a 10 on a numerical scale of

0 to 10, with 10 being the highest. The right hip is warm to the touch and tender. Temperature is 100.5°F, blood pressure 140/88, pulse 109, and respirations 22. The primary care provider ordered Vera to receive 2 mg morphine sulfate every hour as needed for pain. A right hip x-ray was also ordered.

Exercise 9-10: *Fill-in*
The nurse suspects Vera of having a _____

Exercise 9-11: *Select all that apply*
The right hip x-ray revealed a complete, comminuted intertrochanteric fracture. What presented risk factors predisposed Vera to this injury?

❏ Falls

❏ Osteoporosis

❏ Age

❏ Bone cancer

❏ Physical abuse

❏ Automobile accident

❏ Smoker

e **eResource 9-8:** To learn more about the risk factors associated with this injury, consult Epocrates Online: [Pathway: http://online.epocrates.com → select the "diseases" tab → enter "hip fracture" into the search field → under the "diagnosis" tab, select "risk factors" and review content]

Exercise 9-12: *Fill-in*
Vera does not understand complete comminuted intertrochanteric fracture. The primary care provider explains:
A complete comminuted intertrochanteric fracture _____

---

e **eResource 9-9:** To support Vera's understanding, the provider uses a mobile device to access Medscape and show her images depicting this type of fracture: [Pathway: Medscape → enter "hip fracture" into the search field → select "Intertrochanteric Hip Fractures" → select "Background" and click on images]

Exercise 9-13: *Fill-in*
The primary care provider has consulted an orthopedic surgeon for Vera's right hip fracture. The orthopedic surgeon has scheduled Vera for an open reduction internal fixation (ORIF). The surgeon explains that an ORIF is

---

Answers to this chapter begin on page 287.

eResource 9-10: To learn more about this surgical procedure, refer to:

■ Medscape on your mobile device: [Pathway: Medscape → enter "hip fracture" into the search field → select "Intertrochanteric Hip Fractures" → select "Treatment & Management" and review content, focusing on "Intraoperative Details." Be sure to view images]

■ Epocrates Online: [Pathway: http://online.epocrates.com → select the "diseases" tab → enter "hip fracture" into the search field → under the "Treatment" tab, select "Tx Details" and review content]

Exercise 9-14: *Ordering*

The nurse knows that several nursing diagnoses will affect Vera's care. Prioritize the following nursing diagnoses from 1 to 4:

_____ Risk for impaired home maintenance related to fractured hip

_____ Physical activity intolerance related to fractured hip

_____ Pain related to fracture

_____ Impaired skin integrity related to surgical incision

Exercise 9-15: *Select all that apply*

The nurse knows that Vera is at risk for potential complications having this surgery. The primary care provider explains these potential complications to the patient.

❑ Infection

❑ Bloating

❑ Bleeding

❑ Blood clots

❑ Adverse reaction to anesthesia

Exercise 9-16: *Matching*

Match the term in Column A to the definition in Column B.

Column A	Column B
A. Compartment syndrome	_____ Inflammation within the bone secondary to penetration by bacteria, trauma, or surgery
B. Fat embolism	_____ Circulatory compromise that occurs after a fracture
C. Deep vein thrombosis	_____ Most common complication after surgery or immobility
D. Osteomyelitis	_____ Fat globules are released into vasculature and then travel to small blood vessels
E. Avascular necrosis	_____ Pressure within muscle compartments that compromises circulation

Answers to this chapter begin on page 287.

Exercise 9-17: *Select all that apply*

Vera's surgery was successful. Nursing interventions have been implemented. What types of postoperative interventions are necessary to maintain Vera's right hip function?

❑ Encourage patient to exercise by using the over-bed trapeze

❑ Arrange for physical therapist for ambulation and activities of daily living

❑ Encourage patient to turn, cough, and deep breathe to prevent pneumonia

❑ Discourage patient from getting out of bed to prevent complications

❑ Perform a neurovascular assessment

 eResource 9-11: For information about alternative methods for pain management, refer to AAOS's publication *Alternative Methods to Help Manage Pain After Orthopaedic Surgery:* [Pathway: http://orthoinfo .aaos.org → select "Treatments & Surgeries" on the menu → scroll down and select "*Alternative Methods to Help Manage Pain After Orthopaedic Surgery.*" (NOTE: there is additional information here regarding complementary medicine)]

Exercise 9-18: *Fill-in*

The primary care provider has prescribed oral calcium supplementation, oral estrogen, and oral alendronate sodium for Vera. The nurse educates Vera on the purpose of using these medications as it relates to her healing right hip fracture.

Oral calcium supplements: _____

Oral estrogen: _____

Oral alendronate sodium: _____

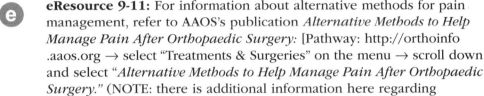 **eResource 9-12:** To reinforce your understanding of these medications, their effects and side effects, refer to Medscape on your mobile device: [Pathway: Medscape → enter "Osteoporosis" into the search field → select "Medications" and review information]

Exercise 9-19: *Multiple-choice question*

Upon discharge to home, the nurse knows Vera understands her home instructions when Vera states:

    A. "I will check my incision site once a week."

    B. "I will watch my incision site for swelling, redness, drainage."

    C. "I do not have to worry about my incision site having a foul odor."

    D. "I will follow my primary care provider's orders for medications only and not exercising."

 eResource 9-13: To reinforce discharge teaching, refer to Medscape on your mobile device: [Pathway: Medscape → enter "Osteoporosis" into the search field → select "Treatment & Management" and review information—focusing on "Dietary Measures," "Physical and Occupational Therapy," "Exercise," and "Long-Term Monitoring"]

Answers to this chapter begin on page 287.

Answers

Exercise 9-1: *Fill-in*

Based on Frances' signs and symptoms, the nurse suspects: **osteoporosis.**

Exercise 9-2: *Select all that apply*

Frances asks the nurse, "What has led to her having this condition?" The nurse explains to Frances risk factors that may lead to osteoporosis.

- ☒ **Family history**
- ☒ **Female**
- ☒ **Age over 60**
- ☒ **Smoking history**
- ☒ **Prolonged immobility**
- ☒ **Postmenopausal estrogen deficiency**
- ❑ Thick, lean body

Exercise 9-3: *Select all that apply*

The primary care provider has ordered laboratory tests to determine the severity of Frances' osteoporosis. What types of laboratory tests are pertinent in ruling out other musculoskeletal disorders?

- ☒ **Serum potassium**
- ☒ **Serum calcium**
- ☒ **Vitamin D**
- ❑ Vitamin A
- ☒ **Phosphorus**
- ☒ **Alkaline phosphatase**

Exercise 9-4: *Matching*

The primary care provider has ordered three diagnostic procedures to determine the bone changes that have occurred.

Match the term in Column A to the definition in Column B.

Column A		Column B
A. Radiographs	__B__	Determines osteoporosis and assesses risk for fracture
B. Quantitative ultrasound	__A__	Reveals low bone density and fractures

Column A	Column B
C. Dual energy x-ray absorptiometry	__C__ Measures bone mineral density in wrist, hip, and vertebral column

Exercise 9-5: *Multiple-choice question*
To minimize further damage or risks of osteoporosis, the nurse would recommend which of the following foods for Frances?
A. Bread/fish—NO, these do not have the calcium needed.
B. Chicken/oranges—NO, these do not have the calcium needed.
C. Milk/yogurt—YES, these are foods that contain calcium.
D. Oatmeal/rice—NO, these do not have the calcium needed.

Exercise 9-6: *Select all that apply*
The primary care provider has prescribed Premarin 0.625 mg daily, calcium carbonate 500 mg twice a day, vitamin D 800 IU daily, and Fosamax 10 mg daily for Frances. What side effects do these medications have in common?
☒ **Headache**
☒ **Nausea**
❑ Slow heart rate
❑ Sore eyes
☒ **Vomiting**
❑ Poor appetite

Exercise 9-7: *Select all that apply*
The nurse knows Frances' care will comprise which nursing diagnoses?
☒ **Activity intolerance**
❑ Imbalanced nutrition: more than body requirements
☒ **Risk for falls**
☒ **Acute pain**

Exercise 9-8: *Fill-in*
Frances is concerned about having fractures with her diagnosis of osteoporosis. The nurse explains to Frances that fractures are **the leading complication of osteoporosis.**

Exercise 9-9: *Select all that apply*
The nurse knows what interventions are important for Frances with the diagnosis of osteoporosis.
☒ **Use safety equipment**
☒ **Educate the importance of regular, weight-bearing exercises**
☒ **Reinforce the need to consume dietary calcium food sources**
❑ Educate on taking calcium before eating
☒ **Remove throw rugs in home, adequate lighting, clear walkway**

Exercise 9-10: *Fill-in*
The nurse suspects Vera to have a **hip fracture.**

Exercise 9-11: *Select all that apply*
The right hip x-ray revealed a complete, comminuted intertrochanteric fracture. What presented risk factors predisposed Vera to this injury?

☒ **Falls**

☒ **Osteoporosis**

☒ **Age**

❑ Bone cancer

❑ Physical abuse

❑ Automobile accident

☒ **Smoker**

Exercise 9-12: *Fill-in*
Vera does not understand complete comminuted intertrochanteric fracture. The primary care provider explains: A complete comminuted intertrochanteric fracture **is a fracture that has fractured through the bone. The bone has shattered into several pieces and it is located at the trochanter of the femur.**

Exercise 9-13: *Fill-in*
The primary care provider has consulted an orthopedic surgeon for Vera's right hip fracture. The orthopedic surgeon has scheduled Vera for an open reduction internal fixation (ORIF). The surgeon explains that an ORIF is **open reduction, which is the correction and alignment of the fracture, and internal fixation, which is the stabilization of the fracture with the use of screws, plates, pins, or wires.**

Exercise 9-14: *Ordering*
The nurse knows that several nursing diagnoses will affect Vera's care. Prioritize the following nursing diagnoses from 1 to 4:

      4   Risk for impaired home maintenance related to fractured hip

      3   Physical activity intolerance related to fractured hip

      1   Pain related to fracture

      2   Impaired skin integrity related to surgical incision

Exercise 9-15: *Select all that apply*
The nurse knows that Vera is at risk for potential complications having this surgery. The primary care provider explains these potential complications to the patient.

☒ **Infection**

❑ Bloating

☒ **Bleeding**

☒ **Blood clots**

☒ **Adverse reaction to anesthesia**

Exercise 9-16: *Matching*

Match the term in Column A to the definition in Column B.

Column A		Column B
A. Compartment syndrome	__D__	Inflammation within the bone secondary to penetration by bacteria, trauma, or surgery
B. Fat embolism	__E__	Circulatory compromise that occurs after a fracture
C. Deep vein thrombosis	__C__	Most common complication after surgery or immobility
D. Osteomyelitis	__B__	Fat globules are released into vasculature and then travel to small blood vessels
E. Avascular necrosis	__A__	Pressure within muscle compartments that compromises circulation

Exercise 9-17: *Select all that apply*

Vera's surgery was successful. Nursing interventions have been implemented. What types of postoperative interventions are necessary to maintain Vera's right hip function?

☒ **Encourage patient to exercise by using the over-bed trapeze**

☒ **Arrange for physical therapist for ambulation and activities of daily living**

☒ **Encourage patient to turn, cough, and deep breathe to prevent pneumonia**

☐ Discourage patient from getting out of bed to prevent complications

☒ **Perform a neurovascular assessment**

Exercise 9-18: *Fill-in*

The primary care provider has prescribed oral calcium supplementation, oral estrogen, and oral alendronate sodium for Vera. The nurse educates Vera on the purpose of using these medications as it relates to her healing right hip fracture.

Oral calcium supplements: **Provide raw material for bone formation**

Oral estrogen: **May stimulate osteoblasts to lay down new bone**

Oral alendronate sodium: **Inhibits the bone reabsorbing capabilities of osteoclasts**

Exercise 9-19: *Multiple-choice question*

Upon discharge to home, the nurse knows Vera understands her home instructions when Vera states:

A. "I will check my incision site once a week."—NO, this should be done more often.

B. **"I will watch my incision site for swelling, redness, drainage."—YES**

C. "I do not have to worry about my incision site having a foul odor."—NO, this is a concern.

D. "I will follow my primary care provider's orders for medications only and not exercising."—NO, both have to be followed.

10

Nursing Care of the Patient With Infectious Diseases

Rhonda M. Brogdon

Unfolding Case Study #47 ▪ Ernest

Ernest is a 66-year-old patient who has come to the emergency department (ED) complaining of fatigue, weakness, aching in his back, dry cough, nasal congestion, and occasional shortness of breath. He states, "I just started feeling bad all of a sudden." He rates his discomfort in his back a 4 on a numerical scale of 0 to 10, with 10 being the most uncomfortable. His health history is positive for hypotension, cerebral vascular accident without deficits, and chronic obstructive pulmonary disease. Ernest's vital signs are temperature 101.6°F, pulse 108, respirations 22, and blood pressure 100/50.

Exercise 10-1: *Fill-in*
Based on Ernest's signs and symptoms, the primary care provider suspects:

_____

Exercise 10-2: *Fill-in*
What signs and symptoms does Ernest present to suspect this diagnosis?

1. _____
2. _____
3. _____
4. _____
5. _____
6. _____
7. _____

The primary care provider (PCP) has ordered a chest x-ray, a pulse oximetry check, oxygen at 2 L/min nasal cannula, and a nasopharyngeal (nasal swab) test for influenza. The PCP knows the nasopharyngeal (nasal swab) test will detect influenza.

Exercise 10-3: *Fill-in*
The nasopharyngeal (nasal swab) test is a:

_____

_____

 eResource 10-1: To reinforce your understanding of diagnostic influenza tests, refer to Medscape on your mobile device: [Pathway: Medscape → enter "influenza" into the search field → select "Diagnostic Influenza Tests" → select "Collection and Diagnostic Methods" and click on Tables. Be sure to review other information as well, particularly "considerations"]

Exercise 10-4: *Fill-in*
Ernest is told that influenza is _____

_____

Ernest does not understand how he contracted influenza (flu).

Exercise 10-5: *Select all that apply*
The primary care provider explains to Ernest that influenza can be contracted by:

❑ Infected blood contact

❑ Touched infected objects

❑ Cough from infected person

❑ Sneeze from infected person

 eResource 10-2: To help Ernest understand how he contracted influenza, refer to:
■ Medscape on your mobile device: [Pathway: Medscape → enter "influenza" into the search field → select "Diagnostic Influenza Tests" → select "Collection and Diagnostic Methods" and click on Tables. Be sure to review other information as well, particularly "considerations"]
■ Show Ernest the video, *What Is Influenza?*
http://youtu.be/bNfU1K-VbDs

Ernest was admitted into the hospital with the diagnosis of influenza and was ordered to be on droplet precautions.

Exercise 10-6: *Multiple-choice question*
The nurse understands that droplet precautions require:

    A. A special ventilation room

    B. Fluid-resistant surgical masks

    C. N-95 respirator masks by visitors

    D. Room door to remain open during lunch

THIS IS NOT VALID

Exercise 10-7: *Select all that apply*

Personal protective equipment that is required for hospital staff include:

❑ Single-use disposable gloves

❑ Fluid-resistant surgical mask

❑ Protective face shield (eyewear/goggles)

❑ N-95 respirator masks

Ernest was ordered to receive Tamiflu 75 mg twice a day for 5 days and intravenous fluids. He was also encouraged to drink fluids to help keep him hydrated.

 eResource 10-3: To reinforce your understanding of Tamiflu, refer to the following resources on your mobile device:

  ▓ Epocrates: [Pathway: Epocrates → enter "Tamiflu" into the search field and review information]

  ▓ Skyscape's RxDrugs: [Pathway: RxDrugs → enter "Tamiflu" into the search field and review information]

  ▓ Medscape: [Pathway: Medscape → enter "Tamiflu" into the search field and review information]

Ernest has begun to feel better. He is afebrile and no longer has the aches he was experiencing upon admission. He states, "I have energy to do my daily walks." Ernest is anxious to go home.

 eResource 10-4: As the nurse plans for Ernest's discharge, the nurse reviews the following material:

  ▓ Centers for Disease Control and Prevention's (CDC's) Seasonal Influenza (Flu) information: www.cdc.gov/flu/

  ▓ Screening Questionnaire: www.immunize.org/catg.d/p4066.pdf

  ▓ CDC Publications: www.cdc.gov/vaccines/pubs/vis/default.htm

The nurse assessed that Ernest did not have his influenza vaccine when reviewing his chart. The nurse knows that Ernest should receive the influenza vaccine.

Exercise 10-8: *Select all that apply*

What indicators does Ernest have that qualify him to receive the influenza vaccine?

❑ Age over 65

❑ History of chronic obstructive pulmonary disease

❑ Complaint of fatigue and weakness

❑ History of cerebral vascular accident

❑ Fever of 101.6°F

 eResource 10-5: The nurse consults the American College of Physicians (ACP) recommended vaccinations to help keep Ernest healthy, for which she has downloaded the ACP Immunization Advisor (ACP-IA) "app" onto her mobile device (http://goo.gl/NZQJB): [Pathway: ACP-IA → select "find" → enter "age" and "condition" (Note: There are no special considerations for Ernest.) → select "Show Vaccines"]

Answers to this chapter begin on page 299.

The nurse explained to Ernest the benefits of receiving the influenza vaccine. Ernest asked the nurse, "What is the difference between the two types of influenza vaccines?"

Exercise 10-9: *Fill-in*

Fill in the difference between the two types of vaccines.

     1. Inactivated: _____

     2. Live, attenuated: _____

Exercise 10-10: *Select all that apply*

The nurse knows that some patients cannot receive the influenza vaccine. This may consist of patients who are:

❑ Allergic to eggs

❑ Reaction to previous influenza vaccine

❑ Positive for Guillain-Barré syndrome

❑ Renal dialysis patients

❑ Pediatric patients

Exercise 10-11: *Select all that apply*

The nurse knows that Ernest understands the side effects of receiving an influenza vaccine (flu shot) by stating he may have:

❑ Low-grade fever

❑ Abdominal pain

❑ Soreness, redness at injection site

❑ Swelling at injection site

❑ Aches

e **eResource 10-6:** To provide supplemental instruction and reinforce the information being provided to Ernest, the nurse uses a mobile device to access CDC Mobile: [Pathway: http://m.cdc.gov → "Diseases and Conditions" → "Seasonal Flu"]

Exercise 10-12: *Fill-in*

The nurse knows there are preventable ways of decreasing Ernest's chances of contracting influenza. Some ways are:

1. _____

2. _____

3. _____

4. _____

5. _____

Answers to this chapter begin on page 299.

eResource 10-7: For more information about prevention of influenza, refer to Epocrates Online: [Pathway: http://online.epocrates.com → select the "diseases" tab → enter "influenza" into the search field → select "Seasonal influenza" → under the "treatment" tab, select "prevention" and review content]

eResource 10-8: To help Ernest understand why he needs to have a flu shot every year, the nurse shows him the following video, *Influenza: Get the (Antigenic) Drift:* http://youtu.be/ug-M1nIhfIA

Unfolding Case Study #48 ▨ Lambert

Lambert is a 45-year-old patient who had received a tuberculin skin test (Mantoux test) 48 hours ago. He presented to the emergency department (ED) with a complaint of redness and swelling at the injection site. He also complained of a persistent cough, loss of appetite, and fatigue. The nurse assessed erythema that was greater than 5 mm and induration greater 10 mm from the injection site. Upon this assessment, the nurse knew Lambert had a positive tuberculin skin test and may be positive for tuberculosis.

Exercise 10-13: *Select all that apply*
What other signs/symptoms are evaluated for active tuberculosis?

- ❏ Bloody sputum
- ❏ Weight gain
- ❏ Night sweats
- ❏ Fever
- ❏ Weight loss

eResource 10-9: To reinforce your understanding of the clinical manifestations of tuberculosis, refer to:
- ▨ Medscape on your mobile device: [Pathway: Medscape → enter "tuberculosis" into the search field → select "Clinical Presentation" and review content]
- ▨ Epocrates Online: [Pathway: http://online.epocrates.com → select the "Diseases" tab → enter "tuberculosis" into the search field → select "Tuberculosis (pulmonary)" review "Key Highlights" and "History" → "Exam"]

The primary care provider (PCP) has ordered sputum specimens for acid-fast bacilli (AFB) smear times three, a chest x-ray, and airborne precautions (respiratory isolation) for Lambert.

Answers to this chapter begin on page 299.

Exercise 10-14: *Fill-in*

The AFB smears will tell the primary care provider:

_____

_____

 eResource 10-10: To learn more about diagnostic procedures for tuberculosis, review:
- Medscape on your mobile device: [Pathway: Medscape → enter "tuberculosis" into the search field → select "tuberculosis" → select "Workup" and review content]
- Epocrates Online: [Pathway: http://online.epocrates.com → select the "diseases" tab → enter "tuberculosis" into the search field → under the "Diagnosis" tab, select "tests" and review content]
- The Merck Manual: [Pathway: www.merckmanuals.com → select "Merck Manual of Diagnosis and Therapy" → enter "tuberculosis" into the search field → select "tuberculosis" → select "Diagnosis" and review content]

Exercise 10-15: *Multiple-choice question*

Lambert cannot believe he may have tuberculosis. He asked the nurse, "How could I have contracted tuberculosis?" The nurse correctly explains:

   A. "Tuberculosis is an infectious disease that usually attacks only healthy people."
   B. "Tuberculosis transmission is by inhalation of droplets from an infected person."
   C. "Tuberculosis is an infectious disease that only attacks the lungs."
   D. "Tuberculosis transmission is by exhalation of droplets from an infected person."

 eResource 10-11: To learn more about causes of tuberculosis, review Medscape on your mobile device: [Pathway: Medscape → enter "tuberculosis" into the search field → select "tuberculosis" → select "Overview" and review content in "Background" and "Epidemiology"]

Exercise 10-16: *Select all that apply*

Lambert's AFB sputum smears were positive for mycobacterium. Lambert has already been placed on airborne precautions (respiratory isolation). What does this mean for Lambert and the hospital staff?

   ❑ Staff to wear N-95 respirator mask
   ❑ Positive air pressure room for patient
   ❑ Negative air pressure room for patient
   ❑ Patient to wear N-95 mask when being transported

Answers to this chapter begin on page 299.

Exercise 10-17: *Fill-in*
Lambert does not understand the reason for airborne precautions. The nurse tells Lambert that airborne precautions are: _____

_____

> **eResource 10-12:** For more information, consult the University of North Carolina Hospital's *Understanding Isolation Precautions*: http://goo.gl/3zBYP

Exercise 10-18: *Fill-in*
The primary care provider has ordered a medication treatment regimen for Lambert. What main four medications are important in the successful treatment of tuberculosis?

1. _____
2. _____
3. _____
4. _____

Lambert is started on this multi-medication regimen.

Exercise 10-19: *Multiple-choice question*
Which of the following instructions should the nurse give Lambert in regard to rifampin (Rifadin)?

    A. "Watch for changes in your hearing."
    B. "The color of your urine may turn orange."
    C. "Take vitamin B_6 daily."
    D. "You may have vision changes."

> **eResource 10-13:** To reinforce your understanding of the medications used to treat tuberculosis, refer to Medscape on your mobile device: [Pathway: Medscape → enter "tuberculosis" into the search field → select "Medication" → select "Antitubercular agents" and review content]

Exercise 10-20: *Select all that apply*
Which medications have to be observed/monitored for hepatoxicity?

    ❑ Isoniazid
    ❑ Rifampin
    ❑ Pyrazinamide
    ❑ Ethambutol
    ❑ Streptomycin

> **eResource 10-14:** To reinforce your understanding of the above medications, their effects and side effects, refer to the following resources on your mobile device:
> ▪ Epocrates: [Pathway: Epocrates → enter "Isoniazid" into the search field and review information. Repeat with the other medications]

Answers to this chapter begin on page 299.

■ Skyscape's RxDrugs: [Pathway: RxDrugs → enter "Isoniazid" into the search field and review information. Repeat with the other medications]

■ Medscape: [Pathway: Medscape → enter "Isoniazid" into the search field and review information. Repeat with the other medications]

After Lambert was in the hospital for 4 weeks, three more AFB sputum smears were completed. The AFB sputum smears came back negative and Lambert's chest x-ray was clear and airborne precautions were discontinued.

Exercise 10-21: *Multiple-choice question*
Lambert asked how often he would have to get a tuberculin (TB) skin test. The nurse correctly replies:

A. "No, you should not get a TB skin test because it will remain positive."

B. "Yes, you should get a TB skin test every year."

C. "Yes, you should get one every 2 years."

D. "Yes, you should get a TB skin test every 3 months."

Exercise 10-22: *Select all that apply*
Upon discharge from the hospital, the nurse knows what type of education is imperative for Lambert.

❑ Practice good hand hygiene

❑ Adhere to medication regimen

❑ Practice respiratory etiquette

❑ Continue with follow-up care

❑ Sputum samples are needed every 2 months

eResource 10-15: To supplement the discharge teaching provided to Lambert, the nurse provides the following pamphlet, *Staying on Track With TB Medicine:* http://goo.gl/So5LF

Answers

Exercise 10-1: *Fill-in*

Based on Ernest's signs and symptoms, the primary care provider suspects: **influenza.**

Exercise 10-2: *Fill-in*

What signs and symptoms does Ernest present to suspect this diagnosis?

1. **Fatigue**
2. **Weakness**
3. **Aching in back**
4. **Dry cough**
5. **Nasal congestion**
6. **Fever**
7. **Shortness of breath**

Exercise 10-3: *Fill-in*

The nasopharyngeal (nasal swab) test is a:

Rapid influenza test that provides results within 15 minutes or less. It is 50% to 70% sensitive for detecting influenza and approximately greater than 90% specific.

Exercise 10-4: *Fill-in*

Ernest is told that influenza is an acute viral disease that is spread through droplet exposure.

Exercise 10-5: *Select all that apply*

The primary care provider explains to Ernest that influenza can be contracted by:

❑ Infected blood contact

☒ **Touched infected objects**

☒ **Cough from infected person**

☒ **Sneeze from infected person**

Exercise 10-6: *Multiple-choice question*

The nurse understands that droplet precautions require:

 A. A special ventilation room—NO, this is not necessary for droplet precautions.

 B. Fluid-resistant surgical masks—YES

 C. N-95 respirator masks by visitors—NO, this is not necessary for droplet precautions.

 D. Room door to remain open during lunch—NO, it should be shut.

Exercise 10-7: *Select all that apply*

Personal protective equipment that is required for hospital staff include:

☒ **Single-use disposable gloves**

☒ **Fluid-resistant surgical mask**

☒ **Protective face shield (eyewear/goggles)**

❑ N-95 respirator masks

Exercise 10-8: *Select all that apply*

What indicators does Ernest have that qualify him to receive the influenza vaccine?

☒ **Age over 65**

☒ **History of chronic obstructive pulmonary disease**

❑ Complaint of fatigue and weakness

☒ **History of cerebral vascular accident**

❑ Fever of 101.6°F

Exercise 10-9: *Fill-in*

Fill in the difference between the two types of vaccines.

 1. **Inactivated: Is a dead vaccine; the "flu shot" is given by injection with a needle.**

 2. **Live, attenuated: Is a weak vaccine that is sprayed into the nostrils. It is recommended for healthy people ages 2 to 49 years of age who are not pregnant.**

Exercise 10-10: *Select all that apply*

The nurse knows that some patients cannot receive the influenza vaccine. This may consist of patients who are:

☒ **Allergic to eggs**

☒ **Reaction to previous influenza vaccine**

☒ **Positive for Guillain-Barré syndrome**

❑ Renal dialysis patients—NO, compromised patients should have it.

❑ Pediatric patients—NO, pediatric patients are at risk.

Exercise 10-11: *Select all that apply*
The nurse knows that Ernest understands the side effects of receiving an influenza vaccine (flu shot) by stating he may have:

☒ **Low-grade fever**

❑ Abdominal pain

☒ **Soreness, redness at injection site**

☒ **Swelling at injection site**

☒ **Aches**

Exercise 10-12: *Fill-in*
The nurse knows there are preventable ways of decreasing Ernest's chances of contracting influenza. Some ways are:

1. **Practice good hand hygiene**
2. **Practice respiratory etiquette**
3. **Know the signs/symptoms of the flu (influenza)**
4. **Stay home if you are sick with the flu**
5. **Annual vaccination for influenza**

Exercise 10-13: *Select all that apply*
What other signs/symptoms are evaluated for active tuberculosis?

☒ **Bloody sputum**

❑ Weight gain

☒ **Night sweats**

☒ **Fever**

☒ **Weight loss**

Exercise 10-14: *Fill-in*
The AFB smears will tell the primary care provider **results of being positive for tuberculosis. It will detect the mycobacterium in the sputum.**

Exercise 10-15: *Multiple-choice question*
Lambert cannot believe he may have tuberculosis. He asked the nurse, "How could I have contracted tuberculosis?" The nurse correctly explains:

A. "Tuberculosis is an infectious disease that usually attacks only healthy people."—NO, this is not true.

B. **"Tuberculosis transmission is by inhalation of droplets from an infected person."—YES**

C. "Tuberculosis is an infectious disease that only attacks the lungs."—NO, it can attack other systems if left untreated.

D. "Tuberculosis transmission is by exhalation of droplets from an infected person."—NO, it is transmitted by inhalation.

Exercise 10-16: *Select all that apply*

Lambert's AFB sputum smears were positive for mycobacterium. Lambert has already been placed on airborne precautions (respiratory isolation). What does this mean for Lambert and the hospital staff?

☒ **Staff to wear N-95 respirator mask**

❑ Positive air pressure room for patient

☒ **Negative air pressure room for patient**

❑ Patient to wear N-95 mask when being transported

Exercise 10-17: *Fill-in*

Lambert does not understand the reason for airborne precautions. The nurse tells Lambert that airborne precautions are: **the isolation of the airborne pathogen to reduce the risk of the airborne transmission of the infectious mycobacterium agent. Airborne precaution requires a negative pressure ventilated room because the bacteria can spread over long distances if exposed to air.**

Exercise 10-18: *Fill-in*

The primary care provider has ordered a medication treatment regimen for Lambert. What four main medications are important in the successful treatment of tuberculosis?

1. **Isoniazid (INH)**
2. **Rifampin (Rifadin)**
3. **Pyrazinamide**
4. **Ethambutol hydrochloride (Myambutol)**

Exercise 10-19: *Multiple-choice question*

Which of the following instructions should the nurse give Lambert in regard to rifampin (Rifadin)?

A. "Watch for changes in your hearing."—NO, this is not a side effect.

B. **"The color of your urine may turn orange."—YES**

C. "Take vitamin B_6 daily."—NO, this is not recommended; it may cause a drug interaction.

D. "You may have vision changes."—NO, vision is not affected.

Exercise 10-20: *Select all that apply*

Which medications have to be observed/monitored for hepatoxicity?

☒ **Isoniazid**

☒ **Rifampin**

☒ **Pyrazinamide**

❑ Ethambutol

❑ Streptomycin

Exercise 10-21: *Multiple-choice question*

Lambert asked how often he would have to get a tuberculin (TB) skin test. The nurse correctly replies:

A. "No, you should not get a TB skin test because it will remain positive."—YES, skin tests are no longer done.

B. "Yes, you should get a TB skin test every year."—NO, it would be positive.

C. "Yes, you should get one every 2 years."—NO

D. "Yes, you should get a TB skin test every 3 months."—NO

Exercise 10-22: *Select all that apply*

Upon discharge from the hospital, the nurse knows what type of education is imperative for Lambert:

☒ **Practice good hand hygiene**

☒ **Adhere to medication regimen**

☒ **Practice respiratory etiquette**

☒ **Continue with follow-up care**

❑ Sputum samples are needed every 2 months

Bibliography

Berman, A., Snyder, S. J., Kozier, B., & Erb, G. (2008). *Kozier & Erb's fundamentals of nursing: Concepts, processes and practice* (8th ed.). Upper Saddle River, NJ: Pearson Prentice Hall.

Centers for Disease Control and Prevention. (2012a). *HIV/AIDS*. Retrieved from http://www.cdc.gov/hiv/resources/factsheets

Centers for Disease Control and Prevention. (2012b). *Testing & diagnosis*. Retrieved from http://www.cdc.gov/tb/topic/testing/default.htm

Centers for Disease Control and Prevention. (2011c). *Influenza symptoms and the role of laboratory diagnostics*. Retrieved from http://www.cdc.gov/flu/professionals/diagnosis/labrolesprocedures

DaVita. (2012). *Stages of kidney disease*. Retrieved from http://www.davita.com/kidney-disease/overview/stages-of-kidney-disease

Hogan-Quigley, B., Palm, M. L., & Bickley, L. S. (2012). *Bates' nursing guide to physical examination and history taking*. Philadelphia: Wolters Kluwer: Lippincott Williams & Wilkins.

Karch, A. M. (2013). *2013 Lippincott's nursing drug guide*. Philadelphia: Wolters Kluwer: Lippincott Williams & Wilkins.

Lutz, C., & Przytulski, K. (2010). *Nutrition and diet therapy* (5th ed.). Philadelphia: F. A. Davis.

Mayo Foundation for Medical Education and Research. (2012). *Your diabetes diet: Exchange lists*. Retrieved from http://www.mayoclinic.com/health/diabetes-diet/DA00077

Smeltzer, S. C., Bare, B. G., Hinkle, J. L., & Cheever, K. H. (2010). *Brunner & Suddarth's textbook of medical-surgical nursing* (12th ed.). Philadelphia: Wolters Kluwer: Lippincott Williams & Wilkins.

Vallerand, A. H., & Sanoski, C. A. (2012). *Unbound medicine version of Davis's drug guide for nurses* (13th ed.). Philadelphia: F. A. Davis.

Van Leeuwen, A. M. (2011). *Unbound medicine version of Davis's comprehensive handbook of laboratory and diagnostic tests with nursing implications* (4th ed.). Philadelphia: F. A. Davis.

Index

Overdue charge is 10 cents per day,
Including Saturdays, Sundays and holidays.